When Empty Arms Become a Heavy Burden

When Empty Arms Become a Heavy Burden

> *Encouragement*
>
> *for Couples*
>
> *Facing*
>
> *Infertility*

SANDRA GLAHN
and
WILLIAM CUTRER, M.D.

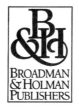

BROADMAN
& HOLMAN
PUBLISHERS

Nashville, Tennessee

Published by Broadman & Holman Publishers, Nashville, Tennessee
Acquisitions & Development Editor: Vicki Crumpton
Interior Design and Typography: TF Designs, Mt. Juliet, Tennessee
Printed in the United States of America
4261-27
0-8054-6127-2
Dewey Decimal Classification: 616.6
Subject Heading: INFERTILITY
Library of Congress Card Catalog Number: 96-34144

Library of Congress Cataloging-in-Publication Data
Glahn, Sandra, 1958.
  When empty arms become a heavy burden : encouragement for
  couples facing infertility / Sandra Glahn, William Cutrer.
    p. cm.
  Includes bibliographical references.
  ISBN 0-8054-6127-2 (pbk.)
  1. Infertility—Psychological aspects. 2. Infertility—Religious
  aspects—Christianity. I. Cutrer, William, 1951–. II. Title.
RC889.G575   1997
616.6'92'0019—dc20
                                                           96-34144
                                                           CIP

97 98 99 00 01 5 4 3 2 1

For all who feel wounds that only the Great Physician can heal.

With love and gratitude to Gary and Jane.

Contents

Introduction

Sandi

"I think I just need to relax," I told the doctor with the kind eyes. I'd just had my annual gynecological examination. "We're putting in long hours with our youth group, I work full-time, and my husband just finished seminary. We've probably been too busy to 'hit it right.'"

"How long have you been trying?" he asked quietly.

"About eighteen months."

He rolled his chair closer. "No, I think maybe it's time to stop 'just relaxing.' There are a few simple things we can try. The pace is up to you."

I had bought into the myth that helped me remain in a state of denial: "If you have trouble conceiving, you just need to relax and you'll get pregnant." It would be several years before I would learn the definition of infertility as the failure to conceive after one year of unprotected intercourse—even if the couple is paying no attention to the monthly cycle. Infertility also includes the inability to carry a child to term. Ninety-five percent of those who fit one of these descriptions have diagnosable medical problems which no amount of relaxing will help. But the good news is that, with treatment, a little over half of those diagnosed as infertile will go on to celebrate a live birth.

I never thought I would join the one in six Americans of childbearing age with fertility problems. I had sworn I would never take my temperature every day, nor would I become "obsessed with getting pregnant" as some of my friends had done. I had never considered myself a "baby" person. So I left the doctor's office and didn't return for another eighteen months.

Finally, we decided to seek further help. Dr. William Cutrer came highly recommended. Not only was he a competent physician; he was also pursuing a master's degree in biblical studies. He had a reputation for being a kind and loving man of God. I wish I could say we hit it off from the beginning, but our doctor/patient relationship got off to a rocky start. This was mostly due to the fact that many of my friends saw him, and I rebelled against what I felt was their "doctor worship." I also felt angry with the process of infertility treatment, and he seemed like a safe place to direct my negative feelings. My husband, Gary, had been loving throughout the entire process, so I didn't want to focus my rage on him, and I knew better than to be mad at God because, as I told myself, *He can do lightning.* So "Dr. Bill," although I liked him, often served as the dart board catching the arrows of bad feelings I hurled in his direction.

Days of Testing

He began by testing Gary, who appeared to have no problem. Most people assume that infertility is the woman's problem, but between 30 and 40 percent of infertility problems reside exclusively in the woman, 30 to 40 percent exclusively in the man, and approximately 30 to 40 percent are shared between husband and wife.

He began to also suspect a structural problem that he felt could have been caused by *in utero* exposure to DES. (DES—diethylstilbestrol—was a medication sold for about thirty years beginning in the 1940s; physicians often prescribed it to reduce the chances of miscarriage. The FDA banned its use after discovering it sometimes caused some structural abnormalities, even cancer, in the children of women who had taken it.)

So I had a laparoscopy. It confirmed no major structural problems and only minimal endometriosis. I spent another year charting my morning temperature, watching my ovaries on the ultrasound screen, taking medication for a mild hormonal imbalance, redefining "spontaneous," and paying multiple medical bills. Gary and I began to feel hurt and annoyed at people who said the wrong thing. We felt helpless in our inability to make long-term plans—I couldn't even buy a pair of jeans without wondering if they would fit in three months. I felt like I was less of a woman. I enjoyed my editing/public relations position with a major insurance company, but I wanted to stay home. My career goals became uncertain. Our pride was injured, our privacy invaded, and our love life became a chore at times. We asked God, "Why us?" and "Why does this hurt so much?"

For the first time, I found I could think of little else besides succeeding in this battle. During those early difficult days, I asked Dr. Bill if he had a support group for his patients. He told me he didn't, but that one of his patients served as a volunteer with a national consumer group for fertility patients. He asked Jennifer to call me. She and I met at a restaurant one day after work, and I found myself laughing more than I had in months. Finally, I had found someone who understood why I felt somewhat insane.

One year after my surgery, I conceived and we were ecstatic. But then I miscarried.

After a break of several months for emotional healing, I reentered treatment. We suspected that a progesterone deficiency had caused my pregnancy loss, so I added daily injections in my hip during two weeks of every cycle. (They gave new meaning to the song, "Twist and Shout.") And I started taking Clomid, a mild fertility drug.

[In the year that followed, Dr. Bill referred me to an endocrinologist.]

I endured another laser laparoscopy and then got promoted to the high-powered fertility drug, Pergonal. This added two more daily shots to my routine. My first cycle on Pergonal resulted in an empty bank account and a second pregnancy, but I lost that pregnancy too. And then another. And then another. (Eventually, we documented eight biochemical pregnancies.)

Decisions, Decisions

In the meantime, our church asked us to lead a support group for infertile couples. I also attended informal support groups where I met many couples experiencing the same pain. Twice my involvement in support groups led me to chair a secular symposium for hundreds of fertility patients and professionals cosponsored by a pharmaceutical company. Dr. Bill taught a session titled "Infertility and Spirituality: Why Me, God?" which was the most popular of the twenty-four workshops.

Our endocrinologist recommended chromosome and antibody analyses, which revealed no problems. He also recommended that Gary use a daily "cooling device," that we affectionately referred to as "Ice Therapy." We began investigating the assisted reproductive technologies (ARTs) such as GIFT and *in vitro* fertilization. About the time we began investigating the moral and financial considerations involved, my sister adopted a little girl. We looked hard at adoption, too, but decided that option was not for us—at least not yet.

Lots of our friends suggested, "Adopt and then you'll get pregnant." But research told us that was another myth; in fact, of those who adopt, only 5 percent conceive. This is the same percentage as those who conceive after deciding not to adopt. Besides, we didn't want to use an adopted child as a means of "fooling ourselves" into getting a biological child. If we chose to adopt, we wanted to open our hearts fully to that child with no other expectations.

Seven years had passed since we had begun "trying." In the meantime, researchers developed a new test for specific antibody problems. We sent in our blood samples assuming the results would come back negative, but we were wrong. We discovered that I am "allergic" to embryos. We felt elated to have a definite diagnosis, even though this condition remains mostly untreatable. There was, however, one therapy we could try. It involved injections of the blood thinner, Heparin, and taking daily doses of baby aspirin.

We felt tired and financially spent, so we took a year off and explored living childfree. At the end of a wonderful year of living a somewhat normal life, we attended a friend's wedding. When we arrived home, Gary said, "I feel depressed."

"Why? Didn't you have a great time?"

"Yes. But did you notice how many of our friends attended with their grown children? For you, it has hurt to see babies; but for me, the pain has come from knowing I will never go camping with my eighteen-year-old."

"So are you saying you want to adopt?"

"I'm saying let's try the Heparin, and if that doesn't work, let's pursue adoption."

Obstetrics in a Different Dimension

We took our time, but after three months I made plans to return to our endocrinologist. Finally, I began to feel motivated to get back into treatment.

Then Dr. Bill invited us to go on a mission trip he was leading to Russia and Belarus. Would we go to Russia or return to treatment?

If we chose to go back into treatment, this was "the night." I asked Gary if he wanted to go to Russia or try to have a baby. He said, "Considering that we don't know, I think we need to wait another month." That sounds pretty reasonable now, but at the time it sounded awful. Waiting one month can seem like an eternity to a fertility patient focused on treatment. Gary kissed me good night, rolled over, and promptly fell asleep. It was not that easy for me.

I had been reading through the Book of Isaiah, so I picked up my Bible and opened it to Isaiah 56. What I read took my breath away:

> The eunuch should not say,
>
> "Because I cannot have children, the Lord will not accept me."

This is what the Lord says:

"The eunuchs should obey the law about the Sabbath.

They should do what I want.

They should keep my agreement.

If they do, I will make their names remembered within my Temple and its walls.

It will be better for them than children.

I will give them a name that will last forever.

It will never be forgotten."

Isaiah 56:3–5 (NCV)

A chill. . . . I had read this in other translations that said, "Because I am a dry reed . . ." and I had never figured out that this passage was speaking to those who could not have children. Now, I'm obviously not a eunuch, but God had used the timeless truth in this passage to speak to me. Other things were more important right now. The next day as I clicked through TV channels, I stopped abruptly on "Star Trek" when I heard this question:

"Why do earthlings consider procreation so important?"

"Because they feel it is their only link to immortality. If they reproduce, part of them lives forever."

That chill again. As a Christian, I have the assurance that I *will* live forever, babies or no babies. *Immortality. I can reproduce in a different realm of reality,* I told myself.

God provided the funds and the time off in miraculous ways, and before long we found ourselves in Russia and Belarus. The following journal entries show the significant events that took place.

October 13. At lunch, Gary and I sat with Lucy and Sergei, a married couple assigned to interpret for us. As we discussed Christianity with them, Sergei said, "It is good that you have brought this information because I may want to become a Christian." I looked for Lucy's reaction, but she didn't respond.

October 14. I was assigned to go door-to-door with Dr. Bill today, and Lucy interpreted for us. After we had seen several peple come to know the Lord, Bill asked Lucy if she had any questions.

"Yes. Why are you trying to change our culture?"

"Every culture has its strengths and weaknesses. We are not here because we think our culture is better; we are here only to share good news." He explained that the gospel was in Russia more than one thousand years before it came to America, and we were only bringing back to the people what the Communist government had taken away.

At the end of the day, Lucy linked her arm in mine. As we walked together, I stopped and asked her what was keeping her from becoming a Christian. She said thoughtfully, "Sandi, I think nothing." So standing there on the Minsk sidewalk, Lucy bowed her head and opened her heart to Him. I told her that even after I left we would see each other again because we'd be together forever in heaven.

There it was. That word. *Forever.* "'It will be better for them than children. I will give them a name that will last *forever,* that will never be forgotten.'"

Reality Check

Within a week of returning home from that trip, Dr. Bill's cardiologist diagnosed him as having a serious heart malfunction and told him he would have to undergo open-heart surgery. During this time, Dr. Bill experienced what it's like to be on the other side of the physician's desk. Since then, he has stopped delivering babies, but he continues to treat fertility patients and devotes many hours to ministry.

Our Heparin therapy failed, so we began to pursue both agency and private adoption. Twice in the past year, we have linked up with birth mothers who changed their minds at the last minute.

It's not over for us, but that's OK. I always hated hearing exhortations to have faith from people who had forgotten how it felt to hurt. I wanted advice from the trenches. We still agonize. We still find suffering a mystery. This week I learned that a woman who was thinking of giving us her baby had an abortion because she got our answering machine instead of a live person when she called. There's too much pain, too many questions. But we also know God is in control, and we can trust Him.

Gary and I have just returned from our third trip to the former Soviet Union with Dr. Bill, where we witnessed more than six hundred professions of faith in one week. Lucy surprised me by meeting me in Kiev this time. She feels thankful that the Lord prevented us from having children when we first wanted them because if He hadn't she never would have known us, nor would she have a personal relationship with the Lord. Her husband and mother have also come to believe in Christ.

Today I number Dr. Bill among my closest friends. It is with pleasure that together we share our vision for helping couples strengthen their spiritual lives and marriages through the agonizing pain of infertility. Even though life is hard, we know God is good, and we have experienced firsthand that He weeps with and comforts those who are hurting.

Dr. Bill

An ordinary day at the office: A quick glance at today's schedule reveals the usual assortment of annual exams, mid-cycle fertility tests, minor gynecological problems, obstetrical visits, and new patient interviews. My office staff notes the nature of the visit beside each patient's name so I can mentally prepare for the day's events. But the word *infertility* never appears. I see real people for real problems and try to avoid labeling individuals as disease processes. I scan this "day sheet" looking for familiar names of patients and families I have known for years. It is a special joy to renew acquaintances and catch up on their lives. When a new patient schedules an appointment for the expressed purpose of discussing infertility, my staff allots additional time. They recognize the depth and detail of discussion ordinarily required to begin a logical evaluation of this complex problem. As a matter of personal preference, I have asked them never to schedule these appointments consecutively because of the time and emotional energy expended by all. Yes, these visits can be stressful from my side of the desk, too, because expectations run high, and feelings are intense.

Often a fertility problem surfaces as a casual remark or question at the end of the routine physical examination. Experience has taught me to approach even the suggestion of concern in this volatile area with the utmost of patience and sensitivity. We may have to sacrifice the office schedule or, ideally, schedule another appointment when we can include the spouse. However, many patients want me to reassure them and give an instant diagnosis which, unfortunately, is impossible. Most who initially come to talk about fertility tend to be overly optimistic, denying the potential seriousness of their problem. Occasionally a patient will arrive with an aggressive, "This is my problem; this is what I need; this is what you will do" attitude. Fortunately, this is rare. Once adversarial feelings develop or basic trust erodes, the close cooperation necessary for a healthy doctor/patient relationship becomes difficult.

The full scope of the infertility evaluation requires both art and science. Diagnostic tests involve anatomy, endocrinology, and function. The order and rapidity of tests may vary, but most practitioners can competently assess and direct therapy if they are committed to their patients and current in their training. As partners respond to detailed questions about their medical and personal histories, they provide many clues about their marital health. As the investigation continues, spiritual issues often surface. I enjoy the "infertility" part of my practice because of its complexity and diversity.

God has permitted us, as clinicians, to understand many of the difficulties involved in His miracle of conception. Thus, I work optimistically trying to offer rational therapies. Of course, I thoroughly enjoy it when testing and therapy result in successful pregnancies, but I have learned much from those who have endured the struggle. I have watched many couples grow in intimacy with each other and in grace with God, even when a successful pregnancy never happens. I try to be honest about my capabilities and to make referrals for high-tech interventions in a timely fashion, when appropriate. Infertility is the most challenging and interesting part of medicine for me now. It is also the most emotionally taxing. The highs are incredible when the efforts produce a desperately desired new life from God. The lows are devastating but provide opportunities to minister God's grace to hurting people and so often these same hurting people minister God's grace back to me. Such is the case with my coauthor and dear friend. On mission fields and in medical conferences, Sandi and Gary have walked with me. We have shared joys and sorrows in the work of Christ. Our relationship has stood the test of time and disappointments. I am grateful to God for enduring friendships that grew from a "routine" patient evaluation.

I can recall a broad spectrum of doctor/patient interactions. Initial encounters with patients have ranged from one husband asking me if his "wife is knocked up yet" to those who are so modest as to act as if another immaculate conception is imminent. Many patients have confessed to adding marks on their temperature recordings indicating multiple romantic interludes to convince me their sex lives are active and "normal." It still amazes me—the lengths to which patients will go to create the illusion of the idyllic marriage. Herein lies the challenge . . . what is normal? Being told when to do it, how to do it, and coming for a "performance analysis" creates a distraction at best.

To what extremes can couples reasonably and biblically go to conceive and carry a child? What ethical questions must we ask, and how can we consistently respond when the technology races ahead of our minuscule understanding of God in creation and conception? And, in the midst of the scientific, medically exhaustive evaluation of the couples' most intimate areas, how can we as health-care providers compassionately respond to the incredible pressures each couple faces from family, friends, and even strangers?

How can we begin to understand the pain and suffering of those in therapy? I simply cannot fully understand, although I know the hurt is profound. My wife, Jane, and I struggled, as she is a "DES daughter." Thus, we fought a personal battle against prematurity and death in the days when medication to stop labor proved ineffective. It would be inappropriate to compare struggles to see who suffers the most. I know, however, personally and professionally, the doubts, the dreams, and the despair of desiring children in uncertain circumstances. Our marriage, as well as our faith, built upon twenty-four years is a testimony to the grace of God in trials and triumphs.

My heart, in this writing, is to encourage those in this struggle—primarily to honor the patients I dearly love and wish I had the ability to give a perfect outcome. We have included many of their stories, although we have changed their names. But our aim is also to support the medical team, the pastoral/counseling people, and even the friends and families of those involved with infertility evaluations. We hope to heighten their sensitivity to the variety of issues, the difficult decisions, and the devastating setbacks that so often overwhelm these couples.

We're all from our own little planets.
That's why we're all different.
That's what makes life interesting.

—*Cary Grant in The Bishop's Wife*

Chapter 1

Not Right or Wrong, Just Different:
Men and Women Handling Crisis

"*W*hat's wrong now, Honey? Why are you crying?"

"I started my period today."

"This is really hard on you, isn't it?"

"Uh huh."

"Maybe we should quit all this treatment stuff. We're destroying our savings account, and it's making you an emotional wreck."

"What do you mean? I thought you wanted a baby!"

"I do, but it's not the most important thing in my life."

"Yeah, but you're not the one getting invited to baby showers."

"No, it's more than that. Maybe other things are important to me—one of them is having my wife back. You're a mess. I can't let you keep doing this to yourself."

"But I can't stop wanting a baby."

"I know, but infertility has changed you. It's all you ever talk about. It's all you ever think about. You cry all the time. You don't want to be with pregnant relatives. You stay home from church because you don't like all the 'baby' announcements in Sunday school. It's become an obsession with you. Something has to give!"

"You're always trying to control me. Now you tell me I have to quit treatment when I want a baby more than anything else."

For this couple, differences in perspective resulted in separation and threatened divorce. Fortunately, they are now back together and in counseling, but most of their problems resulted from misunderstanding a simple truth— that men and women are most assuredly different. Neither the female nor the male perspective is right or wrong, nor is one better than the other.

"I find that I always apologize first when making generalizations about differences between men and women," says Shoshanna, who talks with hundreds of infertile couples as a support group volunteer. "It has become politically incorrect to highlight these differences. Yet in the shift from nurture to nature research, we're beginning to realize we're programmed more than we thought we were."

Many of us, mistakenly assuming that men and women approach problems using the same thought paradigm, scratch our heads in wonder when we miscommunicate. Now, after decades of stressing equality, mental health-care providers admit they have overlooked differences between healthy men and women. Of course, not everyone follows the "mold" of masculine/feminine behavior, nor does everyone agree on the origin of these differences. Approximately 15 percent of husbands and wives display communication styles more characteristic of the opposite gender—a normal variation which makes life interesting and counseling a unique challenge. But, in general, we must acknowledge that we are not the same.

These differences manifest themselves in what we do, say, and think. Unfortunately, we fail to appreciate the affect these God-given, unique perspectives have on marital conflict. However, they are all-pervasive and evident, perhaps even before birth. Although we do not recommend *in utero* counseling, we do suggest that understanding is in order.

Chuck and Jan meant to act lovingly toward each other, but they responded in incompatible ways. Chuck did what many husbands do when faced with the stress of infertility—he assumed a "protector, defender" role. In doing so, he wanted to stop treatment. From his perspective, this was the most loving thing to do. By removing his wife from medical treatment, he believed he was choosing the kindest option in difficult circumstances. In fact, he was accepting the loss of not having children in return for doing what he saw as "right" or "heroic." The female typically views this identical scenario—the husband's willingness to stop treatment—as a lack of love or commitment to the "necessary process." When couples misunderstand the unique factors contributing to their responses, the resulting rift can devastate the marriage.

"In the beginning I assumed that John felt the same as I did about the fact that we could not have a baby," writes Sylvia Van Regenmorter in *Dear God, Why Can't We Have a Baby?*

> I was sure that he must be hurting inside as much as I was, that it bothered him when our friends had a new baby, that he deeply sympathized with me in my weary temperature charting and visits to the doctor, and that he understood when I burst into tears for no apparent reason.
>
> In time, however, it became obvious that my assumptions were wrong. John wanted children badly and was very disappointed I did not become pregnant. But I realized that he was not hurting at the depth or with the same intensity that I was hurting. With that realization came anger. . . . Why did he show only lukewarm interest whenever I brought up the subject of our infertility for discussion?[1]

In a 1985 study, 50 percent of infertile women who responded said that their infertility was the greatest burden they had ever borne. Only 15 percent of the men responding said the same thing.[2] One sociologist who personally experienced infertility and studied infertile couples for five years concluded that gender-based differences significantly complicated the infertility crisis. He observed that, in general, "Wives saw their husbands as callous and unaffected by infertility while husbands saw their wives as 'overreacting' and unable to put things in perspective. While wives felt their husbands were unwilling to talk about infertility, some husbands wondered what there was to talk about."[3]

A psychologist who polled men for their responses found that most of them commonly coped with infertility by "ignoring the problem." On a scale of 0-10, with 10 being "in control," the average male felt he rated a "6" in assessing his own emotional response to fertility treatment. When answering the question, "To what degree did you feel your wife was emotionally in control during your infertility experience?" the average man said "3."[4]

One Christian husband, after researching the emotional impact of infertility on women, said, "I didn't feel the degree of upheaval during infertility that my wife did. I had no idea what she really felt until I conducted my studies. Then I realized I had been to her like those in Jeremiah 6:14, who 'healed the wound of My people lightly, saying "Peace, peace," When there is no peace'" (RSV).

Another researcher found that men have similar reactions to infertility as their wives, but these feelings often occur three years after the wives experience them. So some couples can find themselves "out of synch" with each other for several years.[5]

Writing in *Self* magazine, Jan Short reveals how, though undomestic, she found herself learning to sew so she might "deserve" a baby. "Such behavior," she says, "is hard for husbands to understand—whose less vivid responses in turn mystify their wives. Not very emotional to begin with, many men display a special lack of emotion about infertility. When pressed, they may mutter that they're trying to appear strong for us, but we also know that they're simply different. They're men. 'Why Do They Act Like That?' is the number one topic in my support group, where we vent our feelings to one another instead of driving our husbands crazy, thereby hurting our chances of getting them to help us conceive a baby."[6]

Why *Do* They Act Like That?

Not all differences are necessarily innate. Physiology, parental influences, education, temperament, birth order, and cultural conditioning all contribute to the contrast between the sexes. Experts have written entire volumes on each of these. Although the evidence is by no means conclusive, we will explore the ones we consider most significant in the fertility crisis—cultural and background differences, hormones, and brain factors influencing verbal differences.

Cultural and Background Differences

Most little girls start early playing with dolls and hearing their mothers say, "When you have a daughter. . . ." They grow up assuming they will bear children. When women attend social events as adults they typically answer questions such as, "Do you have children?" while men answer, "What do you do?" Women receive baby shower invitations; most men do not. As a result, even women with successful careers usually feel social pressure to bear and raise children. Males receive a different cultural message: "If you have a family, fine. If you have a job, better." These cultural and societal variables play a significant role in establishing foundational thought patterns and processes.

"Boys grow into men without much thought of fatherhood," says Dan Clements, past Chairman of the Board for RESOLVE, Inc., a national infertility support group. "We think a great deal about school, sports, jobs, careers, earning money, and eventually even about girls, but little, if anything about babies and nothing about pregnancy. Never once do we look at pregnant women and imagine that some day that will be us. Never once does watching others fawning over a pregnant woman—kidding her about her weight, touching her stomach to feel for a kicking baby—create imagined thoughts of the future in our minds. We are taught that when we grow up, we get a job and go to work—always outside the home."

"American women grow up thinking of motherhood as a central—if not *the* central—role in their lives," says one researcher. "While many men also want to become parents, theirs is no 'fatherhood mandate' with the same force and intensity as the 'motherhood mandate.' Since parenthood is deemed to be more central to women's identities than to men's, it stands to reason that the effects of infertility on identity would be more severe for women. And American women and men are still subject to different sets of expectations regarding attitudes, emotions, demeanor, and behavior."[7]

Though our culture has seen some positive changes, most men with wives of childbearing age grew up in environments in which little boys learned to suppress emotion. Their Little League coaches motivated them early to be independent, strong, self-reliant, competitive, and emotionally restrained. Those who did express fear or grief got tagged "fraidy-cat," "sissy," and "Mama's boy." So, years later when confronted with losses, they have difficulty crying, acting "weak," or seeking support.

Yet, Clements argues,

> It is not insensitivity, nor is it necessarily that men are taught not to show their emotions that causes men to feel differently than women about infertility. The emotions that surround infertility are emotions associated with loss. For men who see their primary role in life as working outside the home, the loss related to infertility is the loss of a secondary role, that of being a father, but for women it is the loss of a primary role, that of being a mother. In addition, for women there is the loss of the pregnancy experience.
>
> For a man to truly understand a woman's feelings about infertility, he must, I believe, come to envision her feelings in terms of equivalent loss to himself. He

must imagine what it would be like to be unable to work at all—forever. He must imagine this is not being retired, but as being disabled, just getting by financially, but unable to earn or to even think about earning and producing what you would like. What would his family and friends expect of him and what would they think? His partner grew up seeing herself as having at least one primary job called Mommy. And because she is one half of an infertile couple, she is disabled and not permitted to work.

Take a woman with an unfulfilled "motherhood mandate" and pair her with a man who does not instinctively feel the same way she does. *Voilà!* You have the beginning ingredients for marital frustration. Now, add hormonal differences.

Hormonal Differences

By birth the infant male brain bathes in roughly twice the levels of testosterone of its female counterpart. We may jokingly call this "testosterone poisoning," but it really is the way God intended for boys to develop. A little girl receives more than twice the intrauterine estrogen exposure by birth as the male. By puberty, these differences multiply, and male testosterone reaches levels approximately fifteen times that of the female. Meanwhile, she produces ten times more estrogen than he does.

These hormones have numerous effects. Testosterone is partially responsible for sexual differentiation in the embryo, the sex drive, muscle and hair growth, and aggressive behavior in adults. This aggression often causes the male to view fertility treatment as a threat to "my turf, my territory, my wife." This, in turn, may drive him to "protect" her from doctors, pharmacists, therapists, and anyone else he perceives as posing a threat to her happiness and safety.

While women make testosterone, they produce it at much lower levels. Estrogen and progesterone dominate their hormonal environments. Their bodies release them in a beautifully complex, cyclical fashion when compared with the rather straightforward testosterone production in the male. Scholars have studied exhaustively the rhythm of the female hormone production. It has been artificially manipulated—but never conquered. Estrogen stimulates the libido less than the male equivalent of testosterone. It peaks briefly at mid-cycle, when it produces physical changes conducive to conception; it stirs emotional desires gently toward sexual fulfillment. Following ovulation, or egg release, progesterone becomes the dominant hormone. It thickens the cervical mucus, preventing easy passage of sperm. It also prepares the uterine lining to receive the fertilized egg. In addition, it tends to cause bloating, decreased sexual desire and, at times, catastrophic mood swings. Unfortunately, even these observations can be simplistic. Sexual desire is more than a hormonal response, and not all people respond to hormonal changes identically.

Differing hormones create differing needs in men and women. In his book, *His Needs, Her Needs,* author Willard Harley, Ph.D., identifies a man's top marital needs in order of importance as sexual fulfillment, recreational companionship, having an attractive spouse, receiving domestic support, and admiration. He identifies a woman's top five needs as quite different: affection, conversation, honesty and openness, financial support, and family commitment.[8] Husbands, who generally rate sex at the top of the list, usually feel consistent sexual interest in their wives. Years of testosterone dominance have yielded males who are quickly and easily aroused. In great contrast, their female counterparts will focus most on sexual intimacy at mid-cycle, a comparatively small window, with an increased focus during fertility treatment.

Many husbands are not so naive as to miss the obvious— their wives may "seduce" them only at mid-cycle to "make a baby." These men may resent that their partners expect their "services" when required and avoid them at other times. Some husbands have even called themselves egg slaves ("Do I have 'egg duty' tonight?"), robots, and trained seals.

King Solomon's Song of Songs shows us that God's purpose in creating sexual intimacy encompasses far more than mere procreation. He intended physical oneness to express completeness in the marital relationship. When we engage in sex to produce children while disregarding the ongoing, normal physical and emotional needs of our partners, we dishonor God and our marriage commitments. Remember Paul's words: "Let the husband fulfill his duty to his wife, and likewise also the wife to her husband. The wife does not have authority over her own body, but the husband does; and likewise also the husband does not have authority over his own body, but the wife does. Stop depriving one another, except by agreement for a time that you may devote yourselves to prayer, and come together again lest Satan tempt you because of your lack of self-control" (1 Cor. 7:3–5, NASB).

Rare is the couple who abstains to "devote themselves to prayer"; far more common is the husband who feels deprived and the wife who feels used; often during infertility treatment, the husband may feel both deprived and used. In the next chapter, we will address keeping the romance alive during treatment. But for now, we encourage wives whose lingerie drawers have rusted shut take seriously their loving responsibility to meet their husbands' ongoing sexual needs.

As the stress of treatment intensifies, the wife shares her negative feelings with her husband. She looks to him to give emotional support with encouraging statements such as, "I'm sorry you have to go through this," and comforting hugs given without sexual intent. When he hears his wife talk about a negative encounter with a pharmacist, the protective or combat-ready husband may advise her with what to him seems obvious: "Call back and complain. Talk to the manager!" She feels frustrated that he has not provided what she wants; he finds it difficult to continue listening because she has rejected his solution, leaving him feeling useless.

In circumstances such as this, women may find it helpful to specifically ask for what they need. In response to her husband's statement, "I can't solve this problem. What do you want me to do?" one wife gave her husband the following list:

- Tell me you love me and you know I am sad.

- Tell me you know that it hurts me very much as each month passes.

- Tell me how *you* feel about our childlessness.

- Share with me your vision of our child.

- Tell me about conversations you've had with other people about our infertility.

- Tell me how you feel when others' children are around.

- Tell me how you feel about "producing a specimen."

- Squeeze my hand or wink at me when we're in public, and you know something difficult has been thrown at me. Let me know you're there.

- Let me talk when I need to.

- Hold me when I cry.[9]

Verbal Differences

Part of the wife's desire for conversation stems from the fact that God has apparently created her with a greater need to express herself verbally. This theory comes as a result of these observations:

- Men have fewer fibers connecting their verbal and emotional sides of the brain than women. Some researches believe this is why it is typically easier for a woman to talk about her emotions than it is for a man.[10]

- Little girls talk more than little boys; girls use whole words, whereas boys focus more on making sounds (uh, mmm, varoom, harrumph).[11]

- The average man speaks roughly 12,500 words a day (which he has often used up by the time he arrives home); the average woman speaks more than 25,000.[12]

- Most men talk facts; most women talk facts *and* feelings.[13]

Someone has noted that perhaps men think compartmentally, like bureaus with many drawers. They pull out one at a time, giving the open drawer their full concentration. A woman, on the other hand, is more like a ball of yarn. In her world, everything connects. If this is true, infertility intensifies this contrast between the sexes. A wife can think constantly about her fertility problems while also managing a job, a home, volunteer work, and any number of responsibilities.

Meanwhile, the husband usually thinks categorically, with fertility problems (the "infertility drawer") receiving his full, undivided attention much less frequently. As the wife begins to sprinkle her twenty-five thousand words with constant talk of treatment, her husband may grow weary of the subject. The more she shares, the more he pulls back. The more he pulls back, the more she experiences isolation and feels a need to verbalize her pain. Thus, Merle Bombardieri, a social worker, suggests the use of the "Twenty Minute Rule" to help keep infertility from becoming an all-consuming event and to break the pattern of lopsided communications.

> The goal of the "Twenty Minute Rule" is to stop infertility from eating up your entire life as a couple. It forces you to limit the amount of time you talk about infertility in a given evening. Many find that twenty minutes is best. Set the timer or alarm clock, and stop as soon as possible after the timer goes off. This makes stopping your mutual responsibility rather than something the "bad guy" husband imposes on his "poor thing" wife.

> When this technique is applied, she tends to talk less about infertility. She crystallizes her message because it has to be quick or she'll miss her chance. He listens intently because he knows he doesn't have to listen all night. She feels better because she's no longer driving him crazy and because, finally, she feels listened to.

A remarkable fringe benefit for many couples: when she talks less about infertility, he talks more! It turns out that wives are often grieving for two, expressing their husbands' feelings as well as their own.[14]

Understanding why many husbands and wives act the way they do will not change the way they respond, but it will go a long way toward helping partners interpret and appreciate the foreign love-language their counterparts are (or are not) speaking.

Are Differences Good?

Husbands and wives together bring balance and wholeness, unity out of diversity. When God created Adam, He said, "It is not good for a man to be alone." So after spending an exciting day naming all the animals, Adam received the world's first anesthetic. God then fashioned the first woman and, as a grand finale, instituted marriage. He made Adam and Eve with natural and beautiful differences. The full expression of His image became possible as they realized (or actualized) their distinctive personhoods as husband and wife. Marriage is about synergy—the total yields far more than the sum of its parts. When Adam, feeling incomplete, first saw Eve, he yelled, "This is it!" God did not create one sex, but two, when He wanted to reflect His own image.

But why did He make us so different? How much is genetic, developmental, or environmental? We don't know, and we would not presume to speak for Him. But ask yourself, "Do I really want my husband to be just like me?" "Would I be drawn to my wife if she thought the same way I do?" "Wouldn't our relationships bore us if men and women were identical?" Must we make these differences represent inferiority and superiority? Why can we hardly talk about them without someone suggesting that there's an "in" group and an "out" group?

Rather than resenting, we must seek to understand, even enjoy, the differences. Mark's letter to his wife shows how this understanding can look for couples experiencing fertility problems:

Dear Louise,

In the past year, you've had numerous doctor's appointments, hCG and progesterone shots, puzzling temperature fluctuations, monthly disappointments, and nagging questions. Add to that "love" by the calendar, surgery, and a miscarriage in your desire to give us what we both want. It has been a year of sorrow for you. Yet you haven't let this drive a wedge between us; instead, you've responded in a way that draws me to you more than ever.

One of your key contributions in fanning my flames of love this year has been your quiet contentment with the realization that I don't feel or experience things exactly like you do. You love me as I am without trying to conform me to your image.

Some husbands go with their wives to doctor's appointments; many attend support group meetings; lots of them hand thermometers to their sweeties in the morning, and then carefully record daily temperature readings. Though I have done each of these on occasion, I don't do them often—and that doesn't hurt your feelings. If you want to watch a television show about infertility, you don't insist I view it with you. It took longer for me to accept the idea of adoption than it did for you, but you didn't push me.

You haven't handed me a script. You've left my chapter on love open to however I want to write it, and you've received my humble contributions gratefully. I've tried to meet you on an emotional level, which is what I think you want from me more than anything else, anyway. I've held you in the night when you've cried. When I've thought it would help, I've tried to make you laugh. When you've verbalized feelings, I've tried to listen with compassion. I've prayed for and with you. I've tried to be gentle when your hormones have made you, as you say, "wigged out." I hope these things have shown you that, though we experience infertility differently, we're still in this together.

I wish I could make it all better by placing a child in your arms, but that is out of my control. So, in the meantime, I'll do my best to fill them instead.

All my love,

Mark

Another couple, Jim and Torri, have forged a good working relationship during treatment too. Torri, deeply grateful for her husband's support, wrote these words for Valentine's Day:

He has . . .

- . . . never shown any feelings about preferring a "fertile" wife. Nor has he ever made me believe our infertility was my fault.

- . . . never shown anger when I've thrown temper tantrums about everything from a pregnant woman crossing my path to those darn ovusticks!

- . . . seen me on the bathroom floor crying about starting my period, being infertile, another negative pregnancy test, miscarriage . . . and he has never failed to give the "Life's Not Fair" speech, or the "I Love You Just the Way You Are" speech.

- . . . listened to me tell my *same* infertility story to every infertile (or even possibly fertile) person I know without looking bored or tired.

- . . . never complained when I asked him to drive me to the doctor's office during an ice storm, with highways barely passable, to get my Clomid prescription.

- When you have a husband this great, you can't help but want a family with him."[15]

Infertility treatment, a major stress factor, amplifies already perplexing male/female differences. Clearly the biblical directive is to live, husbands and wives, in an understanding relationship based on selfless, sacrificial love. Since men's and women's social, hormonal, and verbal distinctives seem so diverse, we must anticipate and appreciate these gender-related responses to crises. In understanding we can learn to marvel over, even celebrate, our Creator's mystery in making man and woman in His image and then pronouncing them, as one flesh, "very good."

For Further Reading

Harley, Willard Jr., Ph.D. *His Needs, Her Needs: Building an Affair-proof Marriage.* Grand Rapids, Mich.: Baker Book House, 1986. A guide to marital happiness which contrasts male and female needs and provides guidance about how to meet them.

Tanner, Deborah, Ph.D. *You Just Don't Understand: Men and Women in Conversation.* New York, N.Y.: Ballantine Books, 1990. Known for her scholarly research, Dr. Tanner presents in a readable style how men and women engage differently in the world. She writes from a secular perspective with the goal of better understanding and respecting one another.

Zoldbrod, Aline. Ph.D. *Men, Women, and Infertility: Intervention and Treatment Strategies.* New York, N.Y.: Lexington Books, 1992. Written primarily for health-care professionals.

For Couples' Discussion

1. How are you and your spouse different?
2. How do you handle these differences?
3. Do you agree with Dr. Harley's list of needs and their priorities?
4. If not, how would each of you prioritize your needs?
5. Do you ever use sex as a "bargaining tool"?
6. Do either of you have a need you have not expressed? Is there a specific response you would like to see?
7. How much do each of you talk about infertility?
8. Do you think the "Twenty Minute Rule" might be helpful for you?
9. On a scale of 1-10 (1 being well; 10 being badly), how well do you think you're handling infertility? How would you rate your spouse's response on this scale? How do you think your spouse would rate your response?
10. Do you have any thoughts about how you can better support each other through this difficult time?

There are three things that are too amazing for me,
Four that I do not understand:
The way of an eagle in the sky,
The way of a snake on a rock,
The way of a ship on the high seas,
And the way of a man with a maiden.

—Proverbs 30:18–19

Chapter 2

Can We Strengthen
Our Love Life during Infertility?

We need search no further than the Old Testament in the Book of First Samuel to find that gender-related perceptions of infertility haven't changed much. The wife's name is Hannah. Her husband, Elkanah, has two wives. Having to compete with a "co-wife" would be bad enough, but Penninah is fertile; Hannah isn't. In fact, Penninah's presence may be due to Hannah's infertility.

Penninah, evidently resenting Hannah for being Elkanah's favorite, taunts her mercilessly about her inability to conceive. Meanwhile, Elkanah's children by Penninah have probably dulled any longing he might have for children.

As we read the worn pages of this beloved story, we see Hannah crying, refusing to eat, and showing classic symptoms of depression. Her valiant husband, who means to comfort and cheer her, arrives on the scene with all the Mr. Fix-it logic he can muster and pronounces: "Am I not better to you than ten children?" Can't you hear the volume of Hannah's wailing increase?

Thousands of years later, many couples still find themselves baffled and generally polarized over the emotions surrounding infertility. As the same sun can soften wax and harden bricks, so also the same stresses during infertility can have opposite effects on the marital relationship—it can either soften couples or make them hard. They can find their relationship strengthened or torn apart.

Making marriage a top priority during fertility treatment can be difficult. The estimated 50 percent divorce rate tells us there's stress to begin with. Then, considering that infertility turns up the heat on sex and money pressures—the two biggest causes of marital breakup—it should come as no surprise that infertility strains even the healthiest of marriages. One study found a 41 percent increase in conflict between spouses and a significant decline in marital satisfaction when they were diagnosed as infertile.[1] Infertility can bring arguments and dysfunction, even infidelity, and ultimately failure, but there's also hope. Most couples who survive the infertility crisis find their marriages more satisfying afterwards. They have endured a difficult experience together, and the rewards last a lifetime.

Marriage—A Top Priority

Why is marriage so important? In Scripture, the relationship is paramount, taking precedence over any other human relationship, including children. Our challenge is to be a good "half" of this "one." We see the intimacy that God intended within marriage in Genesis 2; the apostle Paul quoted it afresh in Ephesians 5, that is, "two become one flesh." Besides sexual unity and societal recognition of the union, God intends a spiritual oneness brought about by covenant love.

"Today the bond of marriage is seldom highly esteemed," writes Vicky Love in *Childless Is Not Less.* It behooves us to give our best effort to our marriage and get the fullest blessing from it. From the basic unit *may* come offspring. But regardless, marriages make children; children do not make marriages. Thinking realistically, even families who have children must eventually live without them. Babies do not stay little very long. . . . If you and your mate are among those who will never be *procreative,* then be *pro-couple.*"[2]

Some have suggested that God's key purpose in marriage is children, saying, "Genesis tells us God ordained marriage so husband and wife would come together to procreate."[3] But Beth Spring, a former editor for *Christianity Today* and an adoptive parent observes, "In all the Bible's teaching about marriage, there is no suggestion that children are essential. They are a wonderful gift and blessing, and they are the usual result of a man and woman committing their lives to one another in marriage. God's perspective on marriage involves each partner leaving parents, cleaving to one another, and becoming one flesh (Gen. 2:24). That is all it takes to make a marriage. In the desolation of your infertility, you may want to dust off the marriage vows you said to one another and contemplate the meaning of 'In sickness and in health; for richer or for poorer.'"[4]

After diagnosis of a fertility problem, the "infertile" partner can begin to feel guilty, wondering if the "fertile" partner regrets marrying him or her. A superior/inferior attitude can develop. Partners who say, "I married you because I love you, not so I could have children," lay a foundation of security that's so necessary at this stage. None of us can take credit for our eye or hair color, bone structure, or the length of our eyelashes. Conversely, none of us should accept blame for that which we cannot help—in this case, the impaired functioning of our reproductive systems.

So, regardless of which partner receives a confirmed diagnosis, the couple must begin to view infertility as "our" problem rather than "his" or "her" problem. It does, in fact, affect both partners in areas relating to more than their physical bodies. They both experience feelings of loss.

Infertility as a Crisis of Sexuality

A friend of mine (Sandi's) has observed that one reason infertile couples have difficulty sharing their fertility problems with others is because it means admitting they actually have sex. Sex is a fascinating topic when someone else is the subject of discussion. It becomes a little more difficult when it's focused on one's self. Considering all the jokes from insensitive friends ("Let me show you how it's done"), one would think that sexual dysfunction is a significant cause of infertility. It's not. But when it is a cause, the situation is often easily correctable, and infertility can actually be the blessing that forces couples to deal with problems which might otherwise have plagued them for years.

Sexual Dysfunction as a Cause of Fertility Problems

One of my (Bill's) patients and her husband had never successfully completed intercourse because of pain upon entry. They had not sought a physician's help until they began to wonder if they had a fertility problem. Simple evaluation revealed that Susan's hymen, an ordinarily thin membrane covering the vagina, was essentially intact, preventing vaginal penetration. Jonathan and Susan had been married two years, yet they had never had true intercourse. The solution proved easy, and Susan conceived.

Sexual Dysfunction as a Result of Fertility Problems

While sexual dysfunction is on rare occasions a cause of fertility problems, it comes far more frequently as a result. While the rest of the world says, "I'll bet you're having fun trying," the infertile couple knows secretly that what was once fun has become a trial.

Take a couple with a normal, healthy love life and tell them they have to report every "encounter" to a third party. Most will become self-conscious. After reading that the "average" couple has sex 2.5 times a week, they begin to feel they must compete with this statistic to be considered "adequate" or hide that they "outdo" this statistic, lest they be perceived as overly active.

Next, tell them how frequently they must "find each other," and when they must abstain. Tell them they have to "do it" even when they feel angry, tired, ill, or have had a bad day. Remind them that they will fail to accomplish an important goal in their marriage if they ignore this schedule. Remind them, too, that failing to adhere to this calendar will cost them additional health-care dollars. If they have followed instructions to a *T,* tell them their efforts have not worked and that they will have to repeat this behavior month after month, year after year. It can become like homework or a chore. Something once associated with gladness now serves as a reminder of tears and failure. It can provoke anger when one partner has a business trip, works late, or has trouble "getting in the mood."

Research has shown that more than half of all couples with infertility problems experience changes in their love lives:

- 56 percent of couples report a decrease in frequency of intercourse after a diagnosis of infertility.

- Both women (59 percent) and men (42 percent) report a decrease in satisfaction with sex. Women (49 percent) also say they feel less comfortable with their sexuality.[5]

- Sexual difficulties are five times greater in couples with fertility problems.[6]

Pressure can hinder arousal. From the husband's perspective, impotence and premature ejaculation may precede more complex diagnostic testing. Many couples are reluctant to recognize or admit problems in this sensitive area. Some experts estimate that 90 percent of the sexual act is mental. If the husband is having "performance anxiety," a common problem, failure is all but assured. "Failure" at sex or perceived responsibility for the infertility problem is, in many cases, devastating to the male.

The basic anatomic differences in men and women make "sex on demand" less of a pressure cooker for the wife. She can lose her ability to have an earth-shaking sexual experience; she can even go so far as to lose all enjoyment of sexual intimacy. Her difficulty in becoming aroused may even cause muscle tension that makes intercourse painful. (Gel lubricants must be used externally only, as they can interfere with the movement of sperm through the vagina.)

Yet unlike her husband, her lack of interest will have no impact on her ability to conceive.

"Fertility, masculinity and potency are concepts that are often equated," write therapists Cooper and Glazer. "It is understandable therefore, that when a man is given a diagnosis of infertility, his identity as a man suffers a real setback. He can easily feel impotent and emasculated. Sometimes men with no prior history of sexual inadequacy or dysfunction become impotent for periods of time after they learn about their infertility problem. Even when it is the woman who is infertile, her partner can still feel his masculinity is threatened. Some men have the fantasy that if they were really potent, they would be able to impregnate their wives.[7]

Jim's doctor diagnosed him as having a fertility problem. Several months later he had an affair while on a trip to "prove to himself he was a man." The marriage ended in divorce. Cliff's diagnosis left him impotent. He said he was no longer "interested" in sex or his wife, and he refused counseling. Thomas couldn't sustain an erection or reach ejaculation at mid-cycle. He began to physically and emotionally abuse his wife, saying it was her fault he wasn't interested because she was unattractive and unappealing. After she finally conceived, their marriage recovered.

Other men give excuses such as, "I'm too tired," or "too busy." One husband described being with his wife as a reminder "like a trumpet blast," proclaiming he had failed as a man.

Writing for *GQ*, Arthur Ralston tells of the difficulties that developed when his wife's physician told her to come to the office immediately following sex for a postcoital test: "Another far more upsetting problem arose. Or rather, didn't arise. (Sorry, but it makes me feel better to joke about it.) I became impotent. The whole ugly, tedious, embarrassing business finally got to me. As I had feared, it started when we were supposed to redo the postcoital test for Dr. Graham. I just couldn't do it. For hours, I ran through every sexy thought I'd ever had (or hadn't had). We tried different rooms, positions. . . . We went from the bed to the floor to the couch. Shades down, shades up. Nothing. It was like trying to start a fire with damp kindling and soggy matches." He goes on to say, "Even if the Clomid had worked perfectly, it would have taken a miracle or an adulterous act for Alice to get pregnant, because, even after we'd passed on the postcoital test, I *still* couldn't do it. I felt, deep down, that something was broken, as if we'd been raped. Our fundamental privacy had been invaded. It was a performance, in other words, and I just wasn't up for it.

"Now, I like sex. I like sex with my wife. But I don't particularly like sex with my wife when I'm told by the clinician to do it. . . . Horses may be able to do it fine at a stud farm. Not me. I don't feel right when sex is just hydraulics. I feel silly and pressured. . . . It took a month and a half, but, with the help of a friendly sex therapist, I'm glad to report that I got through this downer. Believe me, I wouldn't be writing a story about it if I hadn't."[8]

Often in the course of the infertility investigation, the husband must produce a sperm specimen "on demand" by masturbation. This can create anxiety for the man who hates to acknowledge that he even knows how to do such a thing.

Many offices, recognizing this difficulty, provide "reading" or "viewing material" to assist in this noble quest. Yet for many couples, this adds to the dilemma. What does it communicate to the wife when her husband uses such aids to produce the specimen, either for analysis or insemination? Add to this the all-too-frequent occurrence of midcycle impotence or "failed ejaculation." This same man who may find himself impotent with his wife is able to successfully produce the specimen by fantasizing over pictures of strangers.

What is our responsibility when it comes to our thoughts? Remember, Paul wrote this: "Whatever is true, whatever is honorable, whatever is right, whatever is pure, whatever is lovely, whatever is of good repute, if there is any excellence and if anything worthy of praise, let your mind dwell on these things" (Phil. 4:8).

Jesus equated lust with adultery. If we are to conduct ourselves, even in the midst of infertility, in a manner consistent with Christian beliefs, our thoughts are important.

A man experiencing infertility might benefit from taking photos (Polaroids, for the sake of discretion) or home videos of his wife, if necessary, to produce a specimen. If he is unable to "perform" with her even when not attempting conception, using these may relieve the pressure long enough for him to discover he still has his manhood after all.

"Scripture neither explicitly condones nor condemns masturbation," we read in the Woman's Study Bible notes. "Jesus does not mention it, nor does Paul include it in his list of vile passions (Rom. 1:26–31). Nevertheless, the moral and psychological ramifications of masturbation can prove disruptive to a relationship with God as well as others, particularly in a marriage. Certainly masturbation does not fulfill God's plan for sexual intimacy between husband and wife (Gen. 2:14)." We would agree, encouraging caution here. But motivation is the key: Are my actions demonstrating respect for God and love for my spouse?

Reading the Song of Solomon and some of the Proverbs, we see that God reveals much about our sexual natures and tendencies. In particular, Proverbs 5:18–19 contains specific encouragements: "Let your fountain be blessed, and rejoice in the wife of your youth. As a loving hind and a graceful doe, let her breasts satisfy you at all times. Be exhilarated always with her love."

God created us in His image as sexual beings. He made our needs and desires. He has ordained marriage as the relationship for the fulfillment of these desires and has given us practical guidelines to help us make decisions. This verse in Proverbs, along with many others, allows us to conclude that sexual expression extends far beyond the "mid-cycle" time of fertility. The very use of the words translated "satisfy" and "exhilarate" suggest more than "dutiful mechanical procreative coitus." In fact, we are to "rejoice" in this physical union.

The Bible prohibits fantasizing about or engaging in extramarital, premarital, multiple-partner, and incestuous sex and sex involving animals. This leaves a wide range of "behaviors" for consideration. However, each of us is a product of many factors, including our upbringing, peer group, past sexual history, and education which make us react very differently to variations in sexual activity. The love and respect a believing spouse has for his or her mate will seek only the best for the other. Thus, couples may exercise creativity and imagination without dishonoring or violating each other's convictions.

Participants in a study investigating how women felt changed by the infertility experience revealed that those whose marriages had survived the trauma reported improvements in several areas: communication, dealing with difficult emotional experiences, and self-esteem. Sexual relationships with spouses were very slow to recover, however, and often still served as a painful reminder of infertility.[9] One might wonder if the fact that couples usually have small children—either through conception or adoption—after infertility might also negatively impact their perceptions of the ongoing sexual relationship. Thus they may "blame" tensions on infertility which might better be attributed to the stresses that accompany their new responsibilities. Nevertheless, it's important to correct any destructive patterns that may emerge while still in treatment. Here are some suggestions.

Overcoming Sexual Difficulties

Change the Time, Place, and Positions

If you always begin your "search and destroy babymaking mission" as a last-minute rush at midnight, get up early. If the bedroom holds too many unhappy memories, find the back seat of the car. (We do not recommend that you try this while the car is in motion.) Planning ahead to create a special time together tells your spouse that you want more out of the experience together than simply an opportunity to attempt procreation. After six straight months of dealing with the "ordered sex" of treatment, Carolyn tells of a time when she tried to ease the pressure: "It's tough on both of us. So I bought a dozen white carnations and a pink rosebud. I put the carnations in a path up the stairs with various pieces of clothing that I had been wearing that day. When he came home from work, he was definitely more 'in the mood' than he might have been otherwise. I had the rosebud in my teeth and was waiting for him in our bedroom."

Talk to Someone

If you are exercising destructive coping methods such as substance abuse, verbal abuse, or violence, seek professional help. Get counseling, too, if you're having difficulty overcoming negative conditioning due to painful sex. Otherwise, an understanding friend may be able to offer support. If he or she does not know how to respond, verbalize what you need—just to talk and have someone listen.

Separate Lovemaking from Babymaking

Couples should "have two sex lives without having an affair" says therapist, Linda Hellmann, who explains what she means using the metaphor of two train trips. The first, she says, is an "express train trip" during which you get to your destination as quickly as possible without dawdling around. It's the few frills, low expectations experience (babymaking sex). The second is the back-road car trip, during which you take your sweet time and enjoy the process thoroughly (lovemaking sex).[10]

Couples undergoing artificial insemination each month can sometimes separate "sex" from "babymaking" more easily since intercourse is no longer a requirement for conception. In fact, one couple become so accustomed to artificial insemination at mid-cycle that when their friends achieved a pregnancy via intercourse, they asked, "You mean you conceived by *natural* insemination?"

Talk Honestly Together about Sexual Difficulties, Being Kind and Tenderhearted

On occasion, tests for sperm/mucus compatibility reveal no sperm in the mucus with a man who previously had a normal sperm count. In other words, he has pretended to ejaculate rather than admit to his wife his inability to "perform" under pressure for the postcoital test. If both partners are honest, they can improve their support of each other; if nothing else, they can commiserate about their mutual problem. A spouse might benefit from compiling a list or "book" outlining what he or she finds sexually exciting (leaving, of course, plenty of room for additions and modifications). Working through sexual difficulties during infertility can actually be an opportunity to improve the degree of pleasure you give and receive together through intimacy at other times.

Guard Your Spouse's Privacy

Carrie, whose husband produced insufficient sperm, told her friends publicly, "Jeez, you'd think he could do his little part correctly." If Carrie's husband wasn't already feeling inadequate, her insensitivity no doubt evoked negative feelings. Keep in mind that your partner may feel more self-conscious than you do about infertility. To assure ongoing trust, be sure that if you do share private information, you do so sensitively and with mutual consent.

Maintain a Sense of Humor

"Through all of our trials and tribulations, my wife and I have found that having a sense of humor has helped," shares one husband. "Our jokes have ranged from my portrayal of the mad scientist while reconstituting drugs to trading stories with other infertile couples of the funniest or strangest places we 'did it' (shots, that is). Answers have ranged from airplane washrooms and backseats of cars to the storeroom of a bar—which happened to have a plate-glass window viewing out onto the street."

Linda and Tim tumbled into bed one night feeling exhausted. Linda groaned and announced, "Tonight's the night," dreading her husband's response. Suddenly Tim sat upright and in his best Sergeant Joe Friday voice said, "It was twelve o'clock. The Clarks were in bed. Then suddenly (to the tune of the Dragnet theme): Ov-u-LA-tion. Ov-u-LA-tion time!" They both laughed and managed to muster up some energy. Most "infertility humor" is not the side-splitting stand-up comedy variety. It's dry, even lame, but it's a wonderful way to diffuse tension.

One couple tells about going to cut down Christmas trees one Saturday in December with another couple from church, Bo and Jackie. The wives, in a moment of privacy, discussed the impending insemination scheduled for the next morning. The next day, the infertile couple met their physician at 7:00 A.M., as instructed. Because they were finished at an early hour, they decided to go to church. When they arrived, they ran into Bo, who asked, "Did you get it up?"

"Excuse me?!"

"Did you get it up?"

The couple looked at each other wide-eyed, shocked that someone would ask something so bold, especially in church. It seemed particularly out of character for laid-back, good-old-boy Bo, who knew how painful infertility was for them. As they stood feeling bewildered and wondering how to answer, he spoke again: "And decorated? Did you get it up and decorated?" He was talking about the Christmas tree they had cut; they thought he meant the insemination.

"Oh! Sure. Of course. Looks great! All those lights and everything." They walked away, concealing their laughter.

Keep in Mind That Infertility Has Nothing to Do with Manhood or Womanhood

"I feel like I've been kicked between the legs," says Kevin, who, after receiving a diagnosis of infertility, expressed feeling inadequate and incompetent as a man.

John the Baptist never fathered children, nor did Jesus Christ, the perfect man. They never even married. Yet we recognize them as great men in history. In her book, *I'm Tired of Waiting,* Elisa Morgan points out that the Suffering Servant, Jesus Christ, as described in the Book of Isaiah, is said to have no descendants, a considerable tragedy in the Old Testament.[11] Yet the Bible greatly honors the investment made in "spiritual children." Later in this prophetic chapter, the writer promises that the Messiah "will see His offspring" (Isa. 53:10).

Even though male/female contributions to procreation are sex-specific, the inability to reproduce does not indicate an absence of manhood or womanhood.

Realize You're "Normal"

No one actually fits perfectly the definition of "normal." "Normal" is an average. Still, take comfort in knowing that most people experiencing infertility have sexual difficulties at some point. Bouts of impotence are far more common than most couples realize, but they are usually temporary.

> According to a story from an early Jewish commentary, a couple married for ten years had no children. The husband wanted to give his wife a divorce so she could marry someone else and have children. So he took her to consult with a rabbi. The rabbi strongly opposed the idea and tried to convince them to stay together, but the husband was adamant. So the rabbi suggested that they throw a party to celebrate their separation. The couple agreed.
>
> During the course of the party, the husband who had drunk too much, told his wife, "Choose whatever you consider most precious in this house and take it with you when you return to your father's house to live."
>
> After he had fallen asleep, the woman ordered her servants to carry her husband to her father's house. In the middle of the night, he awoke.
>
> "Where am I?" he wanted to know.

"At my father's house," she replied. "You told me to take whatever I considered most precious to me. You are most precious to me."

Moved by his wife's love, the husband remained with her, and they lived happily ever after.

Can we strengthen our love life during infertility? Of course. And we start by remembering what (or who) is most precious.

For Further Reading

Christian Guides to Sexual Intimacy

Barton, R. Ruth. *Becoming a Woman of Strength.* (Wheaton, Ill.: Harold Shaw Publishers, 1994). See chapter titled, "The Sexual Journey."

Cutrer, William, M. D., and Sandra Glahn. *Developing Sexual Intimacy.* Grand Rapids, Mich.: Kregel Publications, 1997.

Meier, Richard, Lorraine Meier, and Paul Meier. *Sex in the Christian Marriage.* (Grand Rapids, Mich.: Baker Book House, 1988).

Penner, Clifford and Joyce. *The Gift of Sex.* Waco, Tex.: Word Publishing, 1981.

Wheat, Ed, M.D., and Gaye Wheat. *Intended for Pleasure.* (Old Tappan, N.J.: Fleming H. Revell Co., 1977).

For Couples' Discussion

1. Is your marriage relationship more important to you than having children? If not, what steps do you need to take to reprioritize?

2. How has infertility impacted your love life? In terms of frequency? And satisfaction? Are you guarding your spouse's privacy in this sensitive and intimate area?

3. Are you engaging in practices (unfaithful thoughts, pornography, minimizing your spouse's sexual response) you need to confess to God and abandon?

4. Are you holding a wrong view of sex ("It's dirty"; "It's only for procreation") that is keeping you from being the sexually fulfilled creation God intended you to be?

5. Make a list of what your spouse does that's sexually exciting to you. Discuss this together.

Love seeketh not itself to please,
Nor for itself hath any care,
But for another gives its ease,
And builds a heaven in hell's despair.

—William Blake 1757–1827

Chapter 3

Can We Keep Our Romance Alive during Infertility?

I (Bill) gave an assignment to several Sunday school classes in differing age ranges. The men were to "demonstrate" or "communicate" their love to their wives in a unique way, using no duplications, every day for one week. I told the wives to choose one day—that's right, just one day—and do likewise.

I found the results fascinating. I have to admit, I expected the men to be fairly unimaginative, but I thought they would surely meet the minimum requirements of this challenge. However, most of them interpreted the "task" to require giving assorted gifts. So after giving flowers, candy, and balloons, most of the men felt stumped—no poetry, no kind deeds, or service related to home or family. (Their wives reported an overwhelming lack of enthusiasm for their efforts.) One particularly self-assured man interpreted this assignment to require daily lovemaking, varying the positions seven times. (His wife was less than thrilled when he proudly offered his report to the class.)

The wives, on the other hand, demonstrated more insight into the "heart" of the homework. Some baked favorite foods, wore alluring attire or went all out for the "romantic evening" by getting baby-sitters and making reservations. One washed her husband's car; another organized his workroom (a dangerous idea). Admittedly, the wives had only one event to plan. But the interesting phenomenon that played out consistently in each class was this: Upon hearing the assignment, men understood that they should buy a gift and "intimacy" would result (except for the lone soul who thought gift giving was superfluous when his body was such a prize). In contrast, women tended to understand the task of demonstrating and communicating love to involve the giving of themselves and their time.

Regardless of how couples may demonstrate their love, when we say infertility can have a devastating effect on a couple's sex life, we do not necessarily mean to imply that it is going to destroy their romance.

Although the statistics about the sex life of infertile couples look pretty bleak, some news about their relationships is actually encouraging. The same researchers who noted a decline in marital satisfaction also reported that 63 percent of the women surveyed said their husbands had shown a marked increase in emotional support.[1] "Infertility is the best thing that ever happened to our *relationship*," writes one patient. "We have grown very close, because we've had to work toward the same goals."

At a time when "spontaneous" disappears from a couple's vocabulary, they can still find ways to keep the "romance" alive while their "love life" suffers. Thoughtful gestures—a call during the day, delivering a long kiss, surprise notes in a briefcase—all contribute to strengthening both love and romance.

"Romance and infertility? Aren't the two mutually exclusive terms? Generally, but not always," says Colleen Botsios, a fertility patient in Nebraska.

> Two years ago on Valentine's Day, I was feeling about as low as I had ever been. All the basic infertility

workup had been completed and nothing stood out as an obvious impediment to pregnancy. All the minor imperfections of my system had been corrected and my husband's equipment had been poked, prodded and put through numerous dry runs. My surgeon had scheduled the laparoscopy for February 16, and my only escape was to become pregnant during the late January cycle. It was possible. It could work. Why not? I'm not *really* infertile, am I? But my escape from surgery didn't happen. The cycle ended with my period starting on cycle day 23. *Oh great . . . now I've developed a luteal phase defect,* I thought. The roller coaster was at an all-time low for me. I cried a lot.

But then, as always, I regrouped. It was Valentine's Day. Time to be festive and romantic. As long as I was going to die during surgery (my secret fear), I might as well enjoy my last few days on the planet. We had a whirlpool tub that we'd *never* used for fear of what sitting in hot water could do to the sperm. Figuring we had nothing to lose, I cranked up the dial on the hot water heater.

My husband arrived home from work about 6:00 P.M. and I met him in a sexy nightgown, explaining that I had a romantic evening planned. I showed him to the bathroom which was dark except for the votive candles scattered around. The whirlpool was gurgling away in the corner complete with coconut bubble bath and *really* hot water. There were two long-stemmed glasses and a tray of appetizers. He was very pleasantly surprised, and we both slid into the tub to sip our drinks and savor the appetizers. It was heaven. Then, the mood perfect, we began to giggle. The bubble bath had gone berserk and way overproduced bubbles due to the whirlpool action. We were both slowly entombed in bubbles. They were at least two feet above the top of the tub and still coming. I looked over at my husband, and he was completely surrounded except for his face. We were hysterical. I got the camera and captured his "Bubble Man" persona for posterity. We showered to get rid of the bubbles. Then I went and got the dinner I had left warming in the oven, instructing my husband that we were eating in bed. He made himself comfortable; I returned with beef burgundy, asparagus, and poached pears in raspberry sauce. We refilled our glasses and consumed the lovely dinner, enjoying every moment and bite. After dinner, we had some very comfortable cuddling. My husband held me, my head on his chest in contented silence for a few magic minutes. Then he said to me how much he had enjoyed the evening and the dinner. "You're a regular Julia Child . . . less," he said. And again we both laughed until we were exhausted.

Somehow in the special aura of the evening, infertility, though still close, was somehow far away from us and not so overwhelming. There was temporarily some room to cuddle and smile and laugh heartily. There would be lots of other times to cry and be angry and depressed. Tonight was exempt. After all, it was one of my last nights on earth before my expected demise during my upcoming laparoscopy. A last stolen moment of romance and closeness. What a way to go. (P.S. I didn't die during surgery and am still stealing romantic moments with frequency.)[2]

Deep, meaningful times of communication do not always require this much preparation and ambiance; but creating times of cuddling, closeness, and conversation does take some extra effort. Sometimes couples feel so weary of "having to have sex" during treatment that during their "off treatment" times they avoid each other altogether—not just sexually, but also in showing affection and conversing.

So, besides planning special times of physical intimacy, what can couples do to keep the romance alive?

Strengthening Your Marriage

Keep Talking to Each Other

Talk about anxieties, fears, frustrations, hopes, dreams, and feelings of inadequacy. Some of these topics may surface negative emotions, but the goal is not "absence of disagreement." The goal is oneness, which can only come from the understanding that follows honest expression.

How we communicate is as important as the fact *that* we communicate. Making *I* statements instead of *you* statements makes the wording of negative feelings less threatening. For example, "You don't even care about how I feel," could be rephrased: "I feel isolated and alone—like my feelings are unimportant." This communicates the primary emotion, while removing the accusation.

Also, when your spouse is talking, engage in active listening. This can include restating what you hear him or her saying: "So you want to take a break from treatment because you feel like it's too stressful for us financially right now?" This gives the opportunity for clarification if you have misunderstood: "No. I think we need to take a break because this is really stressing us out emotionally, and next month is going to be especially rough for me at work." (A word of caution: Don't overdo it with restating phrases, or your spouse may ask, "Is there an echo in here?")

We make no promises that communicating well will "make it all go away." Sometimes we won't like what we hear; but before we can work out our differences, we have to know clearly what they are. It's normal to feel guilt, anger, envy, grief, sadness, and isolation. An important part of working through these negative emotions is having and giving the freedom to express them. Instead of saying, "Please don't cry," a more sensitive response might be, "Let me hold you while you cry." Instead of saying, "You shouldn't feel that way, Honey," try, "I wish you didn't feel that way, but I can understand why you do." Sometimes wives report that they have told their husbands, "You don't have to cry. Just don't criticize me when I do."

Couples in crisis must refrain from giving in to the temptation to enter the "Suffering Olympics" (not only with each other, but with outsiders, as well). When your wife shares about something that's hard to endure, don't "one-up" her with statements like, "You think that's bad. . . ." If your husband says, "It's humiliating to be handed a cup and told to go in a stall and produce a specimen," a wrong response is, "Yeah? What about me? I had to have surgery. Producing a specimen is the least you can do considering what I'm going through." A more supportive response would be, "I can't imagine being told I had to do that! Thanks for your willingness to endure embarrassment so we can try to have a child." Rather than vying for the gold medal in the "Worst Trials" event, consider entering the "Special Olympics" where, instead of competing, you help each other cross the finish line and everybody wins.

Every relationship has value beyond reproduction. So talk about what you value in your relationship. One husband writes, "Maybe it's good that we fertility patients can't always have sex when we want it—'down' times can force us to spend some well-deserved time talking." Here are some suggestions to get you started:

1. What is the nicest thing my spouse has ever done for me?
2. What have been some of our favorite romantic moments?
3. What leisure activities do we enjoy?
4. In what ways are our personalities alike?
5. In what ways are we different?
6. In what circumstances have those differences proved to be strengths?
7. If we don't have children in the next year, what would we like to accomplish or plan to do together?

Communicate by Your Actions That "We're in This Thing Together"

Part of making this "our" problem instead of "his" or "her" problem might mean going with your husband to "be there" during his difficult test or escorting your wife to her regularly scheduled sonogram. Showing up for doctor's appointments alone month after month can increase feelings of isolation; particularly during the first few inseminations, wives like to have their husbands present. As one wife said, "I don't want my husband to be in another zip code while I'm lying on the table trying to conceive his child." It's comforting to know someone will be with you or waiting for you while you undergo day surgery or a painful procedure.

One wife shares, "It helps that my husband goes with me and hears and sees firsthand what procedures entail." Another adds, "I find that we understand things better when we've both heard the doctor's explanations."

But that's not always possible. Andy, who often accompanied his wife to appointments, realized he would be unable to be with her for their monthly insemination. When he went to the doctor's office to drop off his specimen before she arrived, he left a dozen red roses and a card for her. He asked the head nurse to place them in his wife's dressing room.

So, if you can't be together in person, there are other ways to say "I'm on your team." Solomon expressed the strength of "togetherness" in some of his best poetry: "Two are better than one, because they have a good reward for their toil. For if they fall, one will lift up his fellow. . . . Again, if two lie together, they are warm; but how can one be warm alone? And though a man might prevail against one who is alone, two will withstand him. A threefold cord is not quickly broken" (Eccles. 4:9–12, RSV).

Take Periodic Breaks

Many infertility patients who would snicker at folks who use lucky rabbits' feet or giggle when they hear about people who fear black cats hold to their own hidden superstition. It goes like this: *If you take a break for one cycle, you will lose the only chance you will ever have to conceive.* Nevertheless, couples must have this time off to "recharge" if they're going to endure treatment for the long haul.

"We have taken several 'breaks' during the last ten years whenever the external sources of stress became too demanding," writes one fertility patient, who believes these periods were the key to her emotional stability. Another says, "Last year during a real down time my husband and I went away on vacation to Washington, D.C. We stayed so busy, we thought only of the fun we were having. I felt so relaxed and just enjoyed the time with him. A third adds, "We like to travel, so we refuse to try cycle after cycle. I think that's why my husband and I seem to handle this fairly well. We've done a lot of stopping and starting."

In addition to taking periodic breaks from treatment, find ways to give yourself emotional mini-breaks. For example, order pizza instead of making dinner sometimes. Let the carpet stay dirty for a few more days if you're not up to doing as much housework. Pay someone else to mow the lawn occasionally.

Find Other Outlets for Verbal Needs

Consider joining an infertility support group as a couple or, if your spouse prefers not to go, individually. Remember what we said about women having twenty-five thousand words they need to use up every day? This is a good place for her to use them up without driving hubby nuts. Support group members won't ever tell you, "Relax and you'll get pregnant" or "You're probably trying too hard." Many husbands have breathed a sigh of relief when their wives have found "infertility buddies" and thus no longer depended on them alone for support.

Connecting with sensitive people at church is another possibility. Numerous references to spiritual gifts tell us that God made us to need one another and to depend on one another for encouragement.

Kayley, a support group leader in a large metropolitan church, notes that most church support group leaders begin by saying, "We want this to be a couples' group because we want to emphasize that this is a couples' problem." But as time goes by, if these groups don't emerge into women's groups altogether, most add "female only" times. Some attribute this to male denial; we don't. Women in general seem to have a greater need for verbal expression of feelings—particularly when it touches on issues as deeply sensitive as infertility.

"I could talk all day about infertility and never grow tired of it," says one female patient. "Networking with other fertility patients provides a great way to meet some of those needs; it also gives me an opportunity to watch God use our experience to encourage others." "Sometimes it's hard to support your spouse when you're having a hard time keeping yourself afloat," says Candy. "So we deal with infertility through one part humor, one part faith, and one part outside support."

Respect That Financial Strain Brings Enormous Stress on the Strongest of Marriages

We're not talking about medium bucks here. We're talking about serious money. In any given month, couples can spend from one hundred to twelve thousand dollars or even more on treatment; adoption is now a five-figure investment. Most husbands and wives have to refrain from doing some pleasurable, perfectly acceptable things to "stay the course." It's important when blowing through this kind of cash that both partners share the conviction to press ahead.

But what if you disagree? What if after communicating effectively you find yourself more upset because you discover that you feel differently about how you plan to handle the "what next"? You may find yourselves at odds over how you want to spend the rest of your money, or your lives, for that matter.

Infertility as a Crisis of Unparallel Paths

Part of "keeping the romance alive" during treatment is recognizing and dealing with the often new and usually traumatic experience of "being at different places" in your decision-making and grief processes. Infertility provides a continuous minefield of choices involving important goals, intense emotions, difficult moral and ethical issues, and finances. Among the choices couples must make are how to communicate, how much to confide in family members, how quickly to proceed, and what tests to endure. Add to that how high-tech to go, whether and when to adopt, and if and when to choose a permanent childfree lifestyle. Couples must make these decisions while their emotions may be clouded by intense pain, and they feel out of sync with each other. For each individual, timing will probably differ on every one of these issues, both emotionally and practically. Also, each of these choices bears a differing degree of importance to the husband and wife.

The common side effects of some fertility medications can also complicate matters. When I (Sandi) started taking Clomid, I told Dr. Bill, "This stuff makes me so emotional, I'd probably cry at mall openings."

"That's not so unusual," he said. "I'd probably cry at mall openings too."

"Yeah, but you mean Grand Openings; I mean when they open the doors daily at ten."

After Suzanne started taking Clomid, she experienced hot flashes and increased emotional responses. Then she became depressed and quit communicating with her husband. In the midst of these difficulties, Suzanne and Bob had to try to make major decisions about treatment. Bob, seeing his wife's distressed emotional state, did not want to pursue the more intense Pergonal therapy her doctor recommended. Suzanne felt strongly that she wanted to give it a try.

When couples fall in love they usually don't reach the point of wanting to marry at the same exact moment. Often one needs more time to "come around" than the other. The only solution is to wait and not push. In dealing with the choices involved in fertility treatment, the path to resolution is much the same.

"Will you decide to adopt or will you choose to live child-free?" asks Mickie, a fertility support group leader. "Both partners may not reach the same decision at the same time. Talk to each other about your needs, dreams, and frustrations.

You don't have to agree, but each of you needs to talk openly. If you continue to talk about your feelings, eventually a strange phenomenon will happen . . . one day you'll be talking, and you'll realize that your goals have merged into a single goal—either you'll agree to adopt a child, or you'll agree to live childfree."

What if you find that after years of demonstrating patience you still disagree? At some point you may need to bring in a third party, such as a pastor or therapist, to help you reach a point of mutual satisfaction. In the meantime, here are some suggestions for getting through those "unparallel" times.

Be Patient

We live in a generation that crosses arms and taps feet as we wait for our microwaves to heat dinner. Some people even shoot drivers who prevent them from shaving two minutes off their road time. Often we need to slow down and let time do its healing work. When we first started treatment, I thought we would never consider (or need) high-tech options. As time passed and we read, discussed, and gained more facts about our case, my perspective changed. Initially, my husband felt opposed to adoption; in time, he changed his mind. So often in a crisis such as infertility, we feel we must "make the decision today," when such decision making is actually premature.

"I read a lot more about infertility than my husband does," says Elizabeth, a nurse. "And I network more with other patients. So I'm more familiar with high-tech treatment and adoption stories than my husband is. As a result, I find that I've often thought through many of the issues earlier than he has. Once I realized I needed to give him time to gain and process information, he felt a lot less pressure from me."

Waiting patiently and praying fervently doesn't always mean your spouse will "come around" to your way of thinking. It may mean the opposite. Tracey shares, "My husband and I began talking seriously about what if we couldn't have any more biological children. He opposed foster parenting, saying he didn't want anyone else's problems, and adoption was unaffordable. Through time, I have come to feel the same way he does, and I believe God has something better planned for me."

Refuse to Manipulate

"My husband initially wanted to live without children," says Joan. "So I purposely messed up our birth control and conceived our first child. We now have several children, but the first has been in and out of mental hospitals for most of her life. I have always wondered how much easier life would have been for us if I had waited for the right timing rather than getting a child via deception. I have never told my husband what I did, and I will go to my grave holding that secret. I will probably always wonder if I'm suffering the consequences of my own actions."

Although Joan conceived easily, she faced the same temptation many infertile spouses face—the desire to manipulate when differences about children surface. While we would like to see her extend to herself the same grace God offers, her experience serves as an important reminder that we need to live in a way that leaves us with as few regrets as possible.

"My husband said a definite 'no' to adoption that began our bout with being 'in different places,'" writes a woman who ten years later is an adoptive mom. "We needed to, as they say, 'put all the cards on the table'; we needed to talk about our feelings, our fears, how our lives would change, and what each of us was willing to give. We had to make certain that building a family was what we really wanted, not just what was expected of us. This was no overnight decision. In time I learned that my husband was trying to spare me from the disappointment of failed adoptions. For us, the key was communication. Pressuring another partner into a quick decision will never work in the long run."

That's not to say we can't nudge or encourage. Dana explains, "My husband, who has always left the decisions up to me, suddenly felt agitated with my stopping treatment. The more I kept putting it off, the more he brought it up, which I found quite unusual. He has prodded me in a positive way to get 'back on the wagon.' He says, 'You can't win the Lotto if you don't play.' He's right. So we're back in treatment." We can influence without trying to control or deceive each other.

Communicate, Communicate, Communicate

"My husband is not as interested as I am in finding out different plans of treatment. This is our main fight," says another patient. "After talking and talking, I discovered he really wants children, maybe even more than I do, but he seems indifferent because he doesn't want to upset me and feels unsure about how to approach the subject with me." In the process of communication we often discover that decisions we have interpreted as unkind or insensitive are actually intended for our good.

Denise writes, "I think that a lot of communicating, even arguing, is the key to making our marital relationship stronger. If we choose to leave nothing dormant, to get it all out where we can look at it, there's a lot to wrestle with. So we get frustrated with each other, sometimes even without resolution. But in the end, my husband tells me, 'Life is such an adventure with you.' I've realized through talking with him that his resistance stems not from selfishness but from worrying about what the medications are doing to me. He is afraid of what we might find out five years down the road. Through putting on the brakes, he's been trying to tell me, 'You're much more important to me than having a baby.'"

Sometimes misunderstanding biblical teaching on marital relationships can complicate the issue here. Carla's husband, Larry, mentioned that he would like to stop treatment. So, without further discussion, Carla called the doctor and told him they were finished. She determined to never bring up the subject again if Larry was against having another child. She felt that she was honoring him in this way. Now, eight years later, she still hides while she weeps in the church balcony on Mother's Day and continues to silently agonize over her feelings. Larry remains oblivious to her pain. The apostle Paul compared the husband/wife relationship to that of Christ and the church. In the same way the church is to bring our requests and express our emotions to the Lord, every wife should know that she must graciously and freely express her feelings to her husband, even if they differ from his.

Sometimes couples think Paul meant "if the husband has an opinion, that's what they must automatically choose to do, end of discussion, case closed." Yet the Word clearly states that husbands are to love their wives as Christ loved the church and gave His life for her. Christ's example of selfless sacrificial love again and again demonstrates that there is no place in the Christian home for a ruthless dictator—or even a benevolent one. In areas of difference, Christian couples should seek unity in making decisions together.

"I recently found out that my husband and I are apparently in disagreement as to how far we'd go to achieve our goal," writes Mindy. "Basically, I'll go as far as I need to and he won't go at all. Unfortunately, I found this out at a party last weekend in front of a bunch of other people. I guess I assumed he'd at least back me on any decision I made. I know we don't communicate well when it comes to these problems. Not only am I depressed; I'm depressed and alone."

"Doing what's right," for Mindy, does not mean giving up and passively resigning herself to a life of misery. Nor does it mean to charge ahead regardless of what her husband wants. As she said, they have failed to communicate well. Her greatest priority now must be to focus on restoring their marriage relationship.

Kind statements such as "You're more important to me than having a baby," "Life is such an adventure with you," and "I want you to be happy," effectively build the relationship at a time when self-images may be at an all-time low. So don't just talk to each other. Speak comfortingly!

Feeling "stressed out" over a crisis situation is a *normal* response, and infertility rates pretty high on the stress scale. It takes hard work, self-sacrifice, and right priorities to strengthen the marriage relationship while enduring sexual, financial, and communication crises. But many couples now look back and say, "After infertility, I feel like we can conquer anything together!"

At a time when we often use the words *success* and *achieving pregnancy* interchangeably, it can be easy to feel like "not achieving pregnancy" means "I'm a failure." But even if we do not ultimately conceive or raise children, we can be successes. God defines success not in terms of what we accomplish; rather, He defines it in terms of the transformation we allow Him to make in our lives. To be the marriage partner I need to be, I must first be the person I need to be.

I am a success if I can get through my infertility experience with a greater love for God and my spouse than when I started.

I am a success if, while experiencing infertility, I refuse to stay focused on myself and find alternate ways to reproduce spiritually.

I am a success if I become an educated consumer and treat wisely the physical body God has entrusted to me—without becoming convinced I'm an expert, without self-diagnosing with every therapy I read about, or without giving unsolicited advice to others.

I am a success if I do not elevate fertility to the level of an idol, making it the driving focus of my life, but instead, continually look for ways to "seek first the kingdom of God and His righteousness."

I am a success on some days if, in spite of my lack of "success," I manage to drag myself out of bed, get dressed, and find reasons to be thankful for one more day.

As a physician friend has so eloquently said, "If the couple goes through the whole process holding their marriage together and emerging stronger, they may not have achieved pregnancy, but in life they are a great success story." So keep talking. Ask God to give you the grace to wait well, and be kind to each another.

Suggested Reading

Becker, Gay. *Healing the Infertile Family*. New York, N.Y.: Bantam Books, 1991. Focuses on the social and emotional difficulties couples face in confronting infertility and how to alleviate them.

Rainey, Dennis and Barbara Rainey. *Strengthening Your Mate's Self-Esteem*. Nashville, Tenn.: Thomas Nelson, 1989. Provides Christian perspective on how to build up your partner. Study guide available.

Salzer, Linda. *How Couples Can Cope*. Boston: G. K. Hall Publishers, 1986. Filled with hundreds of quotes and helpful suggestions for couples on dealing with the stress of treatment.

Davis, Michele Weiner. *Divorce Busting: A Revolutionary and Rapid Program for Staying Together*. New York, N.Y.: Simon & Schuster, 1993.

For Couples' Discussion

1. Why is becoming pregnant so important to you?

2. How, if at all, does being infertile affect your view of yourself as a man or woman?

3. What goes through your mind when you're with friends who don't know about your fertility problems?

4. What goes through your mind when you see a baby?

5. What, for you, is the hardest part about not having children?

6. Describe the ways in which this experience hurts you.

7. Does it change you in each others' eyes if you can't have a child?

8. On a scale of one to ten, how much pain are you feeling over your inability to have kids?

9. How are each of you coping with your grief? Do you feel supported by or isolated from each other?

10. Discuss your answers to the questions on page 46.

Chapter 4

Good Grief!
Why Do I Feel Like I'm Going Crazy?

*S*cientists estimate that seventy-four billion people have lived on Earth since its creation. Four billion of these are alive today; but where will they be one hundred years from now? Old Testament writers called Sheol the place of the dead; the Scriptures, speaking metaphorically, say Sheol never utters, "I'm full—so nobody else can die."

Precipitation in its various forms has covered three-fourths of the earth for thousands of years. Yet the ground continues to soak in the dew, the drizzle, and the downpour. Like Sheol, the earth never utters, "I've had enough."

Blazing fires in and around Yellowstone National Park devoured nearly one million acres of forest. It took the heroics of ten thousand civilian and military fire fighters to keep flames from demolishing the entire park. It seems that fire is never satisfied.

God set these natural laws in motion: the grave, the earth, and fire are always unsatisfied. These laws are mentioned in Proverbs 30:15–16, along with another significant generalization: "There are three things that will not be satisfied, Four that will not say, 'Enough': Sheol, and the barren womb, Earth that is never satisfied with water, And fire that never says, 'Enough.'"

Some people observe a childless woman and say to themselves, "She needs to stop baby craving." Would we expect a fire to stop itself? People to stop dying? Rainfall to sit on the surface of the earth? In general, God instilled in women a need to bear and nurture children. So the tears an infertile woman cries simply validate the truth of what God said in Proverbs. Grieving over infertility and longing for that genetic link is normal.

When righteous Hannah experienced infertility, she wept bitterly, felt "greatly distressed," described herself as oppressed, and wouldn't eat. Notice that God does not say to her, "You shouldn't feel that way."

If infertility were an event, couples could grieve the loss and move on; but infertility is a process. Thus, grief may drag on for years. Many have described it as a roller coaster of hope and despair. Psychologists in one study asked infertility patients to rate the stress of infertility among stressful events ranging from 0–100, with the death of a spouse rating 100, divorce at 73, and the death of a close relative at 63. These patients rated the stress of infertility as sixth of 43 on the scale at 59.7. Another study indicates that fertility patients are second only to cancer patients in what they are willing to endure for a "cure."

Some have identified a pattern to the stages of grief in mourning over lost dreams. One woman wrote, "We discussed the grief process in my psychology class. Knowing each step helped me identify my feelings about infertility that seemed so intense each month. Categorizing them helped me to see that each was typical enough that someone had actually documented it as a normal part of coping."

The Stages of Grief

Denial

The first "stage" of grieving is denial. I [Bill] find it interesting and at times exasperating to watch how couples initially respond. Many begin with a form of denial attributing lack of "success" to timing, stress, or other external factors. Rare indeed is the case in which timing alone is responsible, but most couples have a distorted understanding of the basics of physiology and human reproduction. At the other end of the spectrum are those patients who, upon hearing a diagnosis of infertility, become depressed and hopeless before I order the first test. Patients describe their experience with denial as follows:

> *Mary.* When my period started each month, I would tell myself, "It's only spotting" until the flow began. Then I reminded myself that "some women have a period the first month they're pregnant." Maybe I was pregnant, and I wouldn't know for another twenty-eight days. I would memorize what each period was like to see if it was abnormal or different from the ones I'd had for the last fifteen years. When I realized it was just like all the rest, I knew I wasn't pregnant after all. Unfortunately, this denial process took several days, starting a few days before my period when I would tell myself, "I don't feel like my period is going to start. Maybe I won't have one!" I guess the reason I never cried on the first day of my period is because I was denying that it was actually happening.

> *Bobbie.* I felt upset when a member of my church invited us to help lead a group for infertile couples. I told her in no uncertain terms, "I'm not infertile. I'm just having trouble getting pregnant!"

Anger

As couples continue to feel powerless, their frustration level builds. They often begin to express anger toward God, themselves, their spouses, other family members, friends, people with children, their doctors, and pregnant women.

> *Mary.* Anger would follow a few days later and I would ask, "Why did God make this happen again?" I would get angry at myself as well, saying, "If only we'd had sex every day instead of every other day . . ." You can imagine what I said to myself after a friend told us, "The second ejaculate in one night has a higher con-

centration of sperm." I began saying to myself, "If only we hadn't been so tired—we should have done it twice a night this month." I got angry that I had consumed caffeine, Nutrasweet, taken cold tablets, and done all the things my pregnant friends' doctors put on their "forbidden" lists. If only I hadn't done those things, I would have been pregnant. Maybe I had *been* pregnant; then when I drank that hot chocolate, the caffeine killed the baby, and I miscarried—except it happened the same time my period was due, so I never knew it. I felt angry that millions of fourteen-year-old girls could get pregnant after one night at a party; I felt angry that Fertile Myrtle from the office was pregnant; I felt angry, of course, about all the stupid, well-meaning comments I heard.

Ann. I've read that anger turned inward is depression, and anger turned sideways is humor. That must be why I try so hard to see the humor in it all—I have a lot of anger. I told my husband I thought the reason it took so many millions of sperm to find the egg is because none would humiliate themselves by stopping to ask for directions.

Barbara. After a church softball game, my husband and I went out with a friend who mentioned that someone we know is pregnant. He said he could understand that it was hard for me to hear the news, but I should be happy for her. I told him "I am." A few minutes later this was bugging me and I flat out said, "Don't ever challenge me on whether I'm happy for her. Of course I am. I'm just not happy for *me*." I felt compelled to make this clear.

Tracy. I have so much going through my head. I want a baby so much. It hurt to watch that TV special on breast feeding. My poor husband had to take all the crying and yelling today. We haven't been able to do anything for four months, and I'm outraged. The insurance company loves to take their sweet time with approvals. All I do is watch the days go by, knowing that it will be another cycle we'll miss. I tend to blame it all on my husband when there is no one else to blame.

Part of the anger stems from frustration over a seeming loss of control. This loss of control dominates two realms. The first is the "today"—the inability to manage daily schedules and emotions. The second is the future. Infertility makes it impossible to predict the future or to accomplish goals.

> *Julie.* This morning I had planned to attend a seminar, but I can't go because I have to test my urine for the LH surge, which hasn't happened yet. This is so immobilizing. I wonder what working women do when they don't have private offices in which to set up a chemistry lab.

> *Melanie.* I take my chart to my doctor and get a progress report like a student would. Did I fill it out right? Did I have sex right? Did I ovulate well? Did my temperature do what it was supposed to do? Do I get a good grade this month?

Often patients compensate for their "loss of control" by educating themselves with medical information. Arming themselves with data makes it easier to manage their treatment, and it also helps them make informed decisions about when to stop.

> *Katherine.* I was uncertain about my resources, and I craved information. I found every article on infertility I could in the *Reader's Guide to Periodic Literature* and in Christian periodicals. I studied every infertile woman in the Bible. For me, information made it easier to be in control of my treatment (control defined as having an influence over the outcome). I could ask more intelligent questions and not feel so helpless.

Bargaining

From here, couples often move to "bargaining," cutting deals with themselves and with God.

> *Mary.* I tell myself, "I'll quit drinking caffeine forever—that will show that I really want a baby. I'll be preparing my body in the right way to nurture a child." "I'll have sex more," or "I'll have sex less," or "I'll pray daily to show God that I mean business." I thought He

would honor these bargaining tools. I thought He would look down and say, "Wow. She's willing to give up Pepsi. She loves Pepsi! She must be serious about wanting children. OK. I'll let her have a baby now that she'll give up what her taste buds crave." All that just made me feel worse when I didn't uphold my end of the bargain.

Depression

Months of suppressed anger bring depression. This stems both from feeling helpless and the chronic strain of treatment.

Elizabeth. I cried. I was quiet. I lost my appetite. I withdrew from friends and group activities.

Maggie. My biological clock still has a lot of time left, but my mental clock is running down.

Leigh. Infertility has so many emotional triggers— like those TV pregnancy tests with real couples. I have my own pain; I don't need to see it on TV. Besides, you never see anyone get a positive who doesn't want one, like a scared teenager. Sesame Street did a segment on a mom bringing home a newborn. Ouch!

Jill. I hate going to the mall and walking past maternity shops. I used to loathe seeing pregnant women there until someone reminded me that any woman I see might have been through infertility. I could actually shop without falling apart after that. Of course, when I see a pregnant seventeen-year-old, it's hard to convince myself she tried for very long. Anyway, Pampers and pregnancy test commercials drive me to the mute button.

Some depression also stems from feelings of low self-esteem and decreased self-confidence. Fifty-five percent of women surveyed said they felt less self-confident after they learned of their infertility.

Beth. I had to go to work after my appointment. As I drove, big tears welled up in my eyes. I just wanted to head for home and cry. When I got to work, I called my husband and told him what the doctor said. I said, "You must feel like you got ripped off. When you married me, you thought we'd have a family and now you're not getting what you bargained for."

Lara. Perhaps it's so difficult for me to see pregnant women because they provide such a prominent reminder of my failure to naturally do a basic biological function that any other organism on the planet can do, even if it's only one-celled. I just saw a commercial for roach bait, and the actor says that once a roach has sex, it's pregnant for life. I feel so defeated that I cannot even compete with a lousy insect. I cannot perform a function that every creature on the planet can do—except my husband and me.

Stephanie. I try not to let it get me down, but I feel so "defective"—especially when I see other women my age with oodles of kids. It's gotten to a point that my husband and I no longer associate with couples who have children. At our ages (thirty and thirty-three), it's pretty hard to find childless couples.

Barbara. I don't mind being around people with kids, nor do I mind being with kids in general, being that I adore them. But yes, that big belly just does it. It is indeed a sore, in-your-face reminder.

Robyn. You start to doubt your self-confidence during those many miles that stretch on and on. A woman who has been told she cannot bear children starts to wonder and doubt who she is as a woman. It's part of the process of working through a world that you never thought you'd be a part of.

Guilt often accompanies feelings of low self-esteem. This guilt may stem from prior sexual experiences, abortion, and contraceptive methods. Donna writes, "Twenty years ago I had an abortion. Now I am going through the guilt and hurt of something I did years ago. Ironically enough, infertility has struck me with full force. My doctor tells me an infection, complications brought on by my twenty-year secret, may be responsible for my fertility problem."

Others may feel guilty about delaying childbearing. Still others experience guilt for less tangible negative feelings in general: "Many of my friends were pregnant," writes a patient who avoided baby showers. "I didn't want to take away from their joy. With these mixed emotions I was unforgiving of myself for being selfish. I saw my response as less than Christlike. I wanted all my reactions to be the way I perceived a perfect, godly woman to be. I wanted them to flow naturally and remain indefinitely. When they didn't, I thought, 'Maybe that's why God's punishing me.' I had to learn to forgive myself when I didn't react in that perfect Christlike way, because He forgives me. He gives grace. He builds the bridge between who we are and who we want to be in Christ."

All this anger drives many couples to alienate themselves from painful situations, pregnant friends, and those who have made insensitive comments. Soon they feel that there's no one left who understands. They feel isolated. Their sources of outside support diminish, intensifying their need for intimacy at a time when each feels less capable of providing support.

> *Mary.* I'm dreading the baby shower. I'm afraid conversation will turn to dilation, contractions, and LaMaze breathing. I can't relate; I can't participate; I can't even imagine what it feels like.

> *Lara.* I avoided church last Mother's Day, and I skipped two weeks ago because I found out about an infant baptism. In fact, last Sunday I checked the bulletin to make sure there wasn't a baptism next Sunday. There's a newlywed couple in our Sunday school class, and I'm so afraid she will show up in a maternity dress. I'll just lose it right then and there. I hate how this becomes something I focus on so much, but it's just so ongoing.

> *Charlene.* I went to a baby shower this week. It wasn't too bad shopping for a baby gift or even being at the shower, but I don't think I'll go to any after this. Even if I'm OK, I make it harder for everyone around me to enjoy themselves. They expressed so much concern for me that I ended up having to reassure *them* that I was OK.

Lisa. I've been battling depression for some time now. Why is it so important to me that my doctor thinks I'm an OK person? Perhaps because I've had to confide so much in him. I feel exposed.

Lynda. I am generally an upbeat person, and I really hate being bummed. Sometimes it's my downfall because everyone always expects me to be happy and understand things, but sometimes I just feel like crying.

Roberta. It's a hard road, infertility. It has lots of hills and valleys. It's lonely. You travel it with your husband and, hopefully, it bonds you together in understanding, determination, and faith. There are no signs to tell you how many miles you have to go, but only dependence and faith to direct you. You often feel like everyone else is on a parallel road. You want to be on the same road they're traveling, but you're somehow trailing behind, looking over with desires and dreams of joining them as they move forward with their lives. I found myself not going to church on Mother's Day for a few years. I feared the feelings that would surface there; I didn't want to steal joy from someone experiencing her first Mother's Day pregnant or with a little one; then, I have to admit, I wanted to make it easy on myself.

Each month when her period comes, the wife usually feels a deep sense of loss. Yet she tells herself no loss has occurred. It's true that the couple has not actually lost a physical child, but the concept of a baby exists. They also realize they'll have to face at least one more month of tests, waiting, stress, expense, and uncertainty.

Mourning

When we cry, both our emotions and our bodies release tension, and privately sobbing for a lost dream actually provides a positive expression of sorrow.

Keith. It's a lot like when somebody dunks you too long—that deep ache, gripping your throat and then diving to your lungs. If you fight it, flailing and kicking, you might find air. But what if you don't? All that energy burned. The alternative feels a lot like suicide. The only way you can really conserve oxygen is to hold still, to surrender to the one holding you down, praying that he'll show some mercy and let you breathe. My wife and I want a baby real bad; sometimes I see her fighting for breath, flailing, and taking in water. So I jam my hands deep in my pockets, and I squeeze my eyes tight. I pray we don't drown.

Sally. I felt pain so severe that I was certain someone had torn an organ from my body, leaving in its place a gaping wound, a psychological hurt no one could ever see and few would even comprehend as little more than self-indulgence.

Alma. I have no visible injury, no disease, no dear relative or friend to mourn, only a deep wound in my psyche, a hole where a child might have been. To many this seems like a peculiar overreaction. To me and us and those like us, it is neither. It is real. I had built a not uncommon fantasy, but a wish has no form, and everything seems to remind you of it. There are no rituals to guide your mourning, no headstone in a cemetery.

Acceptance

Eventually, couples who have worked through each stage of the process reach the point of acceptance, looking ahead more optimistically to alternatives. They begin to feel increased levels of energy and enthusiasm. Although the pain never disappears, it somehow becomes more manageable as they gain a renewed sense of purpose, even though they realize they may never bear a biological child. Often couples having the most difficulty getting to this stage are those with unexplained infertility and those who have conflict in their marriages or their families.

Mary. Finally, after a week or so, I would accept that I wasn't pregnant this month; I'd have to wait awhile longer to announce a pregnancy to my family. Soon after the acceptance stage each month, it was time to "try again." Even though I experienced the entire grief process each month, I think infertility is a grief process within a grief process. The cycle of grief that comes and leaves every twenty-eight days is part of a larger cycle that kept me continually asking if I would ever be free. The first month I tried to get pregnant, I experienced grief. Yet the larger grief process didn't begin until six months or more after we started "trying." There are still times I say to myself, "I can't be infertile. I feel fine." Sometimes I'm angry that people less prepared to raise kids become parents. Often I make bargains with myself and God. Whereas the twenty-eight-day grief cycle would keep me from seeing friends a few days a month, the larger cycle kept me isolated for years. Acceptance, too, is part of the bigger cycle. I felt a twinge of the greater grief cycle last night. I visited a friend who had just delivered a beautiful boy. I realized I might never experience holding a child who was the reward of two people's love (or two people's work, a doctor and a basal thermometer). The big difference between then and now: no tears, no canceling all social engagements, no promises to do better, no anger at God, my husband, or myself. I must be moving closer to acceptance.

Debbie. I lost my five-year-old son to leukemia. Six months later we began trying again. That was four years ago. I have now put this into God's hands and taken a break, which has done me so much good—I haven't felt this good in years. I guess I went from the pain of losing a child to the pain of infertility, and now I feel like I have my life back.

Karen. I've had two failed *in vitro* cycles, so I understand the pain; but sometimes when going through infertility, it's easy to become so self-absorbed that we can't see anyone or anything else. If one in six couples of childbearing age is experiencing infertility, five of six are not. If I get bent out of shape at church on Mother's Day, why not dwell on the fact that those five in six women deserve to hear a Mother's Day sermon? Or why not spend the day feeling thankful for my own mother?

These comments present infertility in stages with specific sequencing. However, in general, grieving couples do not experience these reactions in the same order. Unique to infertility, the injection of hope at mid-cycle complicates the entire process.

Mary. After the "Honey, it's our day" stage, I would spend the next ten days thinking, "Did I feel something in my uterus?" I would analyze every gas pain and discomfort thinking, "Maybe I'm pregnant—I think I felt the egg implant!" Every time I went to the bathroom I would say to myself, "I must be pregnant. Pregnant women use the bathroom a lot, and here I sit again." Then a few days later ... *splat* ... back into the wall of denial and the grief process when my period would begin.

Linda. I giggle every time I read about someone looking for the almighty "symptom" that will indicate a successful egg/sperm union. I laugh because I have spent so much money on books with symptom lists. Every time we try, I drag them out, looking for the one thing that may indicate success. Unfortunately, there is no one symptom, twinge, temperature, tiredness, or anything else that will tell you what you want to know. The only thing is a blood test or home pregnancy test taken at the appropriate time. Some months I felt every conceivable (no pun intended) symptom in the books, and even made up some strange ones of my own.

Steve Johnson, a therapist and adoptive father, says, "It is unrealistic to list prescribed stages through which each couple should move. But these stages do provide an accurate description of emotions common to most couples dealing with infertility. Rather than viewing these as steps to be accomplished once and for all, it may be more realistic to view these emotions as part of a spiral which diminishes in size over time. One emotion may be more intense at times than at others."

One psychologist, after reviewing the research on chronic disease, disability and illness notes, "Life events appraised as negative, uncontrollable, unpredictable, or ambiguous are typically experienced as more stressful than those not so appraised." For this reason, Aline Zoldbrod, a therapist who works with infertile couples, says, "Thinking in terms of the grief model is not helpful at every stage of coming to grips with fertility problems." She suggests that patients view their infertility as they would a chronic illness, rather than a linear grief cycle. People who believe that they can do something in response to a stressful event appear to adjust better to those stressful events than those without such feelings of control. She suggests monitoring negative thoughts and arming yourself with information to increase feelings of control.[1]

Infertility as a Crisis of Uncertainty

Is uncertainty stressful? Apparently. The British Health Service reported that during the bombing on London in World War II, stress levels in the city, where bombing was constant, increased by 50 percent. In the outskirts of London, where bombing was intermittent and uncertain, the level of stress increased to over 300 percent.

Uncertainty related to infertility keeps couples from "moving ahead" in the absence of a definite beginning and ending. Some have said that infertility is more like mourning someone missing in action than someone known dead. After the bombing of the Oklahoma City Federal building, a husband who had waited several days before receiving confirmation of his wife's death, said, "I actually feel relieved. Now I know for sure. Waiting and not knowing was the worst part."

In the eleventh chapter of Hebrews—that honor roll of heroes of the faith—comes this verse: "They were killed by stoning, by being sawn in two . . . and then were killed with the sword" (Heb. 11:37, Phillips). "Right in the middle of terrible martyrdoms (stoned, sawn asunder, killed) comes this apparently mild little word *tempted by specious promises of release*," notes Author Isabel Kuhn. "It does not seem to match the other sufferings. And yet no mistake has been made. The slow wearing down of the human spirit is a species of torture which the Communists delight to use and have found very productive for their purposes."[2]

In other words, sometimes hope becomes the enemy. According to the writer of Hebrews, disappointment can be as hard to endure as other life crises. The more optimistic a patient is at the beginning of the month, the harder the crash at the end. As Solomon said so well in Proverbs 13:12, "Hope deferred makes the heart sick."

A couple can feel that their relationship has stagnated because their future is paralyzed. Making good long-term decisions becomes impossible. Does she take that promotion, knowing she may be pregnant next month? How can they plan an overseas trip, knowing travel may be dangerous if she conceives? Should he buy her a dress that emphasizes her trim waistline, knowing it won't fit in a few months if this treatment works? Gary and I (Sandi) bought a station wagon in anticipation of our growing family. When the odometer read two hundred thousand miles, we still had no children.

After months—even years—pass, couples can feel they are wasting their lives. The more medical developments they hear about, the longer they find themselves staying at it, eliminating all the possibilities. Uncertainty becomes a way of life.

"Infertiles are like those hamsters who play for hours on a wheel, going nowhere, never getting off," says Mary Martin Mason, in *The Miracle Seekers*. "Around you life spins by—your career, your family, your marriage, your friends—without your participation. "[3]

Within infertility's overall holding pattern is a monthly holding pattern of making adjustments "just in case" you're finally pregnant.

> *Barbara.* Waiting is the hardest. It's been eight days since our IVF embryo transfer. I just want to get it over with so that I know what I'm dealing with, and I can try to live normally again for those brief few weeks before the onslaught of the next IVF. How desperately I ache for a normal life again. That pregnancy test is going to happen . . . and while you wait for it, you put your life on hold and have to act as though you are already pregnant—just in case. The week after embryo transfer, you can't do anything strenuous so that your precious embryos may implant firmly. So for two weeks you have to pretend you're pregnant, being careful, of course, not to get carried away with the fantasy of it all.

Forced to pretend at something you desperately want and then discovering that you really aren't pregnant after all."

Another patient says, "I put aside too many things for 'after I have children' . . . and soon half my life had slipped away while I sat 'on hold.' I was nearing forty, and everything I'd assumed would come naturally wasn't happening. No children, no career. It was easy to feel sorry for myself and look for circumstances to blame."

An old Indian proverb says, "Waiting shreds the spirit; knowing rends the heart in two that it may begin to heal." Infertility means waiting—waiting for those "other plans" to materialize. It's one of many such times—waiting to find the right person to marry, waiting for the right job, waiting to sell a house, or waiting for a payoff after years of hard work. In fact, we spend most of our lives waiting. The Scriptures, especially the Psalms, contain numerous admonitions to wait on the Lord. Abraham waited his entire adult life without ever finding the city God sent him out to find. Hebrews 11 contains long lists of people who "died in faith without receiving the promises" (v. 13). They died waiting. Yet each demonstrated faith in how he or she waited. It seems that God considers *how* we handle the wait as important as "what we're waiting for." Yet we mustn't confuse waiting with passively sitting around, anticipating that God's plan will someday roll around and hit us. Abraham's "wait" involved actively leaving his home and country and heading for the promised land.

"Your father (not my fiancé, yet) made a three-week voyage by sea from San Pedro, California, to Ecuador," writes Elizabeth Elliot, to her daughter in *Let Me Be a Woman.* "[He stopped] at fascinating ports along the way, from which he sent me fascinating letters. He began his study of Spanish in Quito without me. He made his first trip to the jungle where he was later to work. He had his first opportunity to do medical work, his first crack at an unwritten language—all of these were things I myself longed to do, and longed desperately to do with him. 'Let not our longing slay the appetite of our living,' he wrote to me, and those words have helped me very often since. We accept and thank God for what is given, not allowing the not-given to spoil it."[4]

Couples cannot "speed up" their mourning so they can feel better again. As we've said, due to its cyclical nature, infertility fails to fit exactly into the "grief process" model. Thus, as mentioned earlier, some therapists have suggested that we view it more as a chronic illness or as Post-Traumatic Stress Disorder than a clear-cut loss. Resolution becomes less of a goal than adaptation and coping.

Some couples find relief in always planning something they can accomplish or enjoy only if they do not conceive. For example, Jana began working on her master's degree, knowing she would have to drop out of school if she got pregnant. Even though she still had no children several years later, all her friends joyously celebrated her graduation. She had done her best to keep herself "in motion," and now she had something to show for it. Each month when Jana learned medical treatment had failed, she comforted herself saying, "At least I get to stay in school."

How to Cope

One key to dealing with grief is recognizing that it's unwise to try to cope alone. We can't emphasize enough the benefits of connecting with other patients and supportive believers throughout the process.

"Last Monday I met with some other infertility patients at Chili's," Maureen said. "When our waiter asked if we were a special group, we told the truth. Afterward one woman said, 'It's like saying you belong to a hemorrhoid club.' Then she added, 'Hey, don't knock it. We're every high school boy's dream.' Her comment was tacky, but it felt good to laugh together."

Most on-line networks have bulletin board services where patients with computers and modems can "connect." Other suggestions for dealing with negative feelings include the following:

- Identify your feelings and acknowledge your losses. If you repress them, they will find other ways out.
- Accept that grief is a normal response to an abnormal situation.
- Let yourself cry when you feel like it.
- Find a physician team that you can trust. (More on this later.) In most cases, the staff is as important as the physician.
- Listen to worship music and attend worship services.
- Live "one day at a time" and work on enjoying to the fullest other areas of your life.
- Allow yourself a healthy avoidance of some situations which, for now, evoke emotions you can't resolve.
- Arm yourself with the facts, and thus give yourself more control in an uncontrollable situation. Most libraries have databases where patients can access up-to-date medical information.

Finally, remember that you're not alone. As one woman wrote, "Although it often seems that way, there is some reassurance in knowing that you are not the only one who is experiencing these feelings." Others know how you feel. The Lord carries you. *You are not alone.*

Resource Organizations

INCIID (International Council on Infertility Information Dissemination; pronounced "inside")
P. O. Box 91363
Tucson, AZ 85752-1363
520/544-9548
INCIIDinfo@AOL.com
HWWK11E@Prodigy.com
http://www.mnsinc.com/inciid/inciid.html
   International organization that offers medical conferences, fact sheets, a newsletter, and on-line support.
RESOLVE
1310 Broadway
Somerville, MA 92144-1731
617/623-0744

Provides fact sheets, referral, support and advocacy for couples with fertility problems including pregnancy loss.
Ferre Institute, Inc.
258 Genesee Street, Suite 302
Utica, NY 13502
315/724-4348
This organization sponsors conferences, publishes brochures and newsletters, maintains a library, and also administers a genetic counseling program.
Endometriosis Association
8585 North 76th Place
Milwaukee, WI 53223
1-800-992-3636

On-line Sources

On the Internet, you can find infertility and adoption discussion groups (newsgroups) called <alt.infertility> and <alt.adoption>. Also, several World Wide Web sites offer information about infertility and photo listings of children available for adoption. Be aware that many Internet sites, while providing a wealth of information, serve as subtle advertising sources.

For Couples' Discussion

1. Do you feel like the "grief cycle" represents your experience?
2. Which of the emotions described here have you experienced?
3. What, if any, stage or stages of the grief process do you feel like you are currently experiencing?
4. Would you benefit from getting some professional counseling?
5. How can you connect with others who can support you?
6. Are there any situations you can avoid to make it easier on yourself?
7. What can you do to arm yourself with more information?
8. How is infertility impacting your relationship with God? If negatively, how can you restore and/or improve your spiritual walk?
9. Are you regularly engaging in meaningful worship?
10. Read Psalm 139. What does this say about how God sees you and your body? Spend some time telling God how you feel.

Like one who takes off a garment on a cold day,
or like vinegar on soda,
Is he who sings songs to a troubled heart.

—*Proverbs 25:20*

Chapter 5

When Everyone Says
the Wrong Thing

Carol and her husband Tim, a theology professor, have one child. After years of treatment, they have given up trying for a second child. One evening they went to dinner with members from a Sunday school class who were trying to recruit Tim as their teacher. One of them asked Carol, "Do you have children?"

"Yes."

"How many?"

"One. A girl."

"Just one?"

"Yes."

"How old is she?"

"Seven."

The men looked at Tim and popped off with, "I guess we won't ask you to teach on sex."

Tim could teach them more about sex and reproduction, about FSH and LH and hCG and sperm counts, than they could possibly want to know. Yet these men connected his inability to father another child with incompetence in the bedroom and ignorance about sex. People can be so wrong and so insensitive.

I [Sandi] had to laugh recently when I read one of the verses in Job. It seems that the patriarch grew rather tired of hearing his friends' "blame the victim" explanations for why "God was punishing him" (which of course He wasn't). So he said to them, "Surely wisdom will die with you." Can't you just hear his sarcasm? So, it appears that the question of how to respond to people's senseless remarks is a timeless problem.

Every fertility patient deals with it. In fact, whenever I sit in a room full of quiet patients, I've found a quick way to get conversation going. I ask, "Has anyone ever made an insensitive remark to you about your infertility?" At first they give me the "duh" look, which says the stupidity of my question is on par with "Has Oprah ever been on a diet?" After that momentary pause, they all stumble over each other trying to be the first to tell their horror stories. They proceed, one-upping each other with, "You think that's bad? My mother-in-law said . . ." and greeting each story with a chorus of sympathetic gasps.

I know you've heard them all and more. So if we've missed your pet comment, add it to the list. Go ahead. Blow off some steam with us here:

What Others Say

Blaming the Victim

"You can always adopt. Then you'll get pregnant. That happens all the time." (If you'd distract yourself into relaxing with a placebo baby, you'd get the real thing.)

"Just relax." (It's your fault because you're trying too hard.)

"Take a vacation." (A variation on the relaxation myth.)

"Keep a positive mental attitude." (It's probably psychological.)

"Are you sure your doctor knows what he's doing?" (If you'd do a better job of managing your medical care, you'd get pregnant.)

"Aren't you pregnant yet?" (What in the world are you doing wrong?)

"What did you do to make yourself infertile?" (This is too absurd to bother interpreting.)

"You waited too long." (Therefore, you deserve this.)

Minimizing Pain

"You should feel . . ." (Your pain is illogical.)

"You're lucky. You have so many other things going for you." (How ungrateful of you!)

"Are you sure you want kids? You can borrow mine this weekend." (I won't feel your pain because being "funny" is better than being "kind.")

"You're young . . . you still have plenty of time." (You're overreacting.)

"Conception is such a complicated process. It's not surprising you're not pregnant. It's a miracle anybody is." (So why are you so surprised?)

"You've been trying for three years? That's nothing—I have a friend who tried for eight years and finally had a baby!" (You lose the Pain Competition.)

"How can you miss something you never had?" (Think it, but don't say it—"Like your brain?")

"Don't you think it's time to move on?" (Aren't you over this yet?)

"I know exactly how you feel." (One woman heard, ". . . because that's just how I felt when my cat died.")

"At least . . ."

Loss of a twin: "At least you have one of them. Be thankful."

Secondary infertility: "At least you have one child. You should be glad you have one." (How ungrateful of you, again.)

Getting Too Personal

"When do your fertile days fall this month?" (Some etiquette books recommend responding to questions like this with, "Why would you ask a question like that?")

"Have they tested your spouse?"

"Stand on your head after intercourse."

"What did your doctor do to you today?"

Speaking on Behalf of the Almighty

"Maybe God . . .

" . . . is punishing you."

". . . is trying to tell you that you're not ready to be parents yet."

". . . is trying to teach you some lesson."

"The Lord will bless you with a child in His timing."

"You need to just turn it over to the Lord." (Real Christians don't grieve.)

"It must be God's will." (Suck it up and take it, you unspiritual wretch, you!)

"God won't give you more than you can take." (So are you questioning God?)

While some of these may ring with actual spiritual truth, they can smart like a stubbed toe when uttered by well-intentioned "comforters."

Miscarriage and Ectopic Pregnancy

"You know it's for the best."

"The baby was probably deformed—this is nature's way of taking care of it."

"You're young."

"You can always have another."

"At least you know you can get pregnant."

"At least you never knew the baby. It would have been harder if it were five . . ."

Empty Reassurances

"You'll surely have a baby by next Christmas."

"God has to bless you with a biological child—you're such a nice couple."

"I know you're going to have a child. I can just sense it from the Lord."

Innuendo

"Your wife can't get pregnant? I'll help!" (You're inadequate.)

"What? Don't you know how it's done?" (You're ignorant.)
"But aren't you having fun trying?" (Don't be so negative.)

Total Ignorance

"Try artificial insemination. My niece and her husband did that, and twelve years later, she conceived." (I'm not making this up.)

Just Plain Meanness

"Nanny nanny boo boo, I got pregnant first!" (OK, so nobody ever said that, but I *know* she thought it.)

In dealing with these insensitive remarks, we've discovered two kinds of people—those who are trainable and those who aren't. Most people will change, if we help them.

Dealing with Hurtful Remarks

Allow Yourself to Feel Frustrated

"Be angry and sin not," wrote Paul. Furthermore, he went on to say, "Let not the sun go down upon your wrath" (Eph. 4:26). People say stupid things that upset us, and it's OK to feel frustrated, even outraged at times, but one of the Spirit's fruits is self-control. So it seems that we must throw our tantrums in private, yet publicly refrain from decking people, both physically and verbally.

While medical tests of infertility stretch our love and patience, people's tacky comments and unsolicited advice push us to our outer limits of self-control. We must have abundant supplies of self-control to keep from retaliating.

Tell God How You Feel

So often we lick our wounds, calling friends who will help us bash any insensitive brutes who hurt us. Yet the psalmists express their anger, frustration, and pain *to God.* Hannah cried to the Lord in desperation when the other mother in her home continually agitated her with unkind words about her fertility problem. Our Heavenly Father offers a prescription for negative feelings—fervent prayer: "Be anxious for nothing but in *everything* by prayer and supplication with thanksgiving, let your requests be made known to God, and the peace of God which surpasses understanding will guard your hearts and minds in Christ Jesus" (Phil. 4:6–7). God encourages us to bring our feelings to Him and vent them before His throne. Christ knows what it feels like to receive insults from others who don't understand. When we offer our emotions to Him, He sympathizes and promises grace and mercy to help in time of need.

Return "Evil" with Good

One of my mentors says, "Grow in giving away grace." She surprises people by showing them unmerited favor, returning their hurtful words and gestures with kindness. Her thinking comes from a time-tested source: "If your enemy is hungry, give him food to eat; and if he is thirsty, give him water to drink. For you will heap burning coals on his head, and the LORD will reward you" (Prov. 25:21–22). Isn't it interesting that this verse immediately follows the one quoted at the beginning of this chapter—the one about "singing songs to a happy heart"? The two go together, I believe.

Sometimes our kindness will show itself in thoughtful words; at other times, it may mean gently and lovingly correcting error.

So, let's say we've allowed ourselves to feel frustrated, we've taken our emotions to God, and we've vowed to return evil with good. Can't we do something more? Can't we educate the poor buffoons who continue to hurt us? Sometimes.

We can never totally keep people from offering unsolicited advice or criticizing us for grieving, but we can try to help them learn how to support us. Yet it's hard to express to them what we need unless we ourselves can articulate what we want from them. So, what do we want?

What We Want from Others

We Want Them Simply to "Be There"

One of our favorite stories is about a farmer who accidentally ran his John Deere into the ditch while plowing his fields. Try as he might, he failed to get the tractor out. Finally he folded his arms, sighed, and just sat in the cab staring at the ground. His neighbor drove by, saw him sitting there, and got out to help. Realizing his inability to solve the problem, he did the next best thing. He climbed into the cab, folded his arms, sighed, and stared at the ground with his friend.

We have no need for supporters who try to cheer us up by minimizing pain or quoting platitudes; we don't want advice unless we ask for it. We do, however, need to hear that we have good qualities even if we remain unable to reproduce. We want our friends and families to simply climb up into the cab and sit there with us while we're stuck in the ditch.

Silence, a touch, and simple assurances go a long way toward healing: "I'm sorry," "How can I help you?" "I'm here to listen if you want to talk about it," "I feel sad for you," "How are you doing?" "Can I hug you?" and "It's OK to cry."

We Appreciate Those Who Will Enter into Our Pain with Us

The Bible tells us to "weep with those who weep." Verses about God's grace pack a lot more punch coming from the one enduring trials than they do coming from the onlookers. When outsiders say, "Trust God," it feels like they're accusing us of not trusting Him. That robs us of the opportunity to speak of His grace. It's the comforter's job to weep over our pain; it's our job to testify of God's sufficiency. Too often it happens the other way around: the comforters leave us weeping after telling us, "God is sufficient."

During my (Bill's) first year of practice, a couple lost a baby at twenty-three weeks. Feeling at a total loss for words, I sat in silence and wept with them. I was surprised when they later thanked me profusely, saying, "You said just the right words."

"What words?" I wondered.

(Precisely.)

We Need Supporters Who Will Validate Our Sense of Loss

Any statement that includes, "At least . . ." or "You should feel . . ." minimizes the sense of loss couples feel. Even if we make jokes about our infertility, we generally don't appreciate it when others do. For example, we flinch when we hear, "Take my kids this weekend if you want a baby so much." What these parents have intended as humor has minimized our pain. In moments of greatest despair, nothing anyone says helps. At those times our pain will cloud our ability to think straight, and it may be impossible for anyone to "do or say the right thing."

We Want Our Friends to Be "Straight" with Us

I (Sandi) don't want friends to hide the news that someone's pregnant because they're afraid I'll commit suicide or something. That's humiliating. A kinder response takes place in private conversation or, even better, through a note: "Sandi, I know this may be hard for you to hear, but I'm expecting. Call when you feel like it." Or, "We'd love for you to attend Jamie's baby shower, but we'll understand if you decide not to come."

We Need Our Supporters to Have Patience with Us

Our needs and choices change. During the "hope" part of a cycle, I often felt comfortable shopping for baby gifts. Days later when I'd start my period, I'd feel differently. I appreciated friends who flexed with my apparent inconsistency. The entire process of treatment can take years longer than most want to endure with us, sometimes turning their compassion to contempt. We need our loved ones to "suffer long." It feels long to us too.

We Need Them to Be Especially Sensitive at Holiday Time

Most patients loathe Mother's Day (otherwise known as M-Day). Peggy writes, "On Mothers' Day, the minister had just finished his sermon and asked all the mothers to stand up. I didn't like that idea because I knew I would be the only woman left sitting. I knew this would be another incident during which I felt singled out again—left to sit alone. I had grown tired of that feeling. The minister proceeded to tell the mothers how God views them as special because He has blessed them with children. Tears welled up in my eyes as I sat wondering why I wasn't special, wondering why He had singled me out. Why wouldn't God bless me with children? I could only hope no one would see those tears starting down my cheeks. I don't know why I felt like I always had to hide my heartache. I guess I was unsure whether anyone else would understand the extent of it, or maybe I felt my emotions demonstrated a lack of faith."

Another patient writes,

> I can remember the hurtful question of four years ago, "Are you going to bother with a Christmas tree since you don't have children?" Society tells us that Christmas is a family time, a time for giving gifts to children, of ho-ho-ho and fa-la-la, and certainly not a time to reflect on the pain we might be experiencing. But for those of us who claim Christian faith, we must think again about what this time really is for us. And when we strip away the hoopla, we again find the message of hope. Christmas is about a baby, yes. But don't forget that this baby grew up and experienced tremendous suffering for the sake of the world. The meaning of Christmas isn't the tinsel; it is God's gift of love. Perhaps the children's pageant will be too difficult to attend. Perhaps the family gathering will be a painful time . . . but when we go back to the real event that we celebrate, the words of John's Gospel ring out to us: "The light shines in darkness and the darkness cannot overcome it."[1]

We fear sitting there on Mother's Day, feeling left out, totally ostracized. We need friends who understand why Christmas, a holiday which focuses on a birth, makes us cry. We want them to cringe with us when someone says, "Christmas is for the children," knowing that it's not just for kids, but for everyone—for unto *us* a child is born, unto *us* a son is given. Consider our Lord's gracious words to those who shouted insults. Only One with supernatural power could pray, "Father, forgive them for they know not what they do." We have that same power at our disposal. We have only to abide in the One whose accusers nailed His hands and feet to a cross—the One who also said, "Apart from Me you can do nothing."

For Further Reading

Johnston, Pat. *Understanding Infertility: A Guide for Family and Friends.* Order this booklet from Perspectives Press, P.O. Box 90318, Indianapolis, IN 46290-0318. This is a great little resource to give those you consider "trainable."

For Couples' Discussion

1. How might you have been guilty of making insensitive remarks in the past?

2. What have people said and/or done relating to your infertility that you found offensive?

3. Have you taken your complaints to God? If not, take a few moments to do so.

4. Whom do you think would benefit from "being educated" about their well-intentioned but painful remarks? Would you feel comfortable asking your pastoral staff to remember those who are hurting in their Mother's Day and Father's Day prayers?

5. How can you show grace to those who do not deserve it?

6. If there is someone who has been especially sensitive to your pain, take a few moments to write a thank-you note.

*It is better to heal with promises
than to promise healing.*

—Calvin Miller, The Philippian Fragment

Chapter 6

Dealing with the Third Party
in Your Love Life: the Physician

*F*reud supposedly said that whenever a husband and wife make love, six people are present—the couple and both sets of in-laws. In the case of fertility patients, add another—the doctor. Through the course of treatment, Gary and I (Sandi) had three physicians. We often imagined them standing at our footboard, tapping their feet, taking notes, and looking clinical. There's no way around it: infertility introduces a third party into a couple's love life. Because "not having a baby" can be all-consuming, it's easy to expect far too much from this person whose Porsche you're sure you just financed. I wrote the following "Wanted" advertisement after a particularly frustrating encounter with one of my doctors. I needed to remind myself that sometimes my expectations were a little too high.

> **WANTED: Physician.** Must work seven days a week while enjoying a strong marriage and family life. Will attend conferences for professional development, but is always in the office; never takes vacations but cultivates many outside interests and international perspectives so as to be well-rounded and interesting. Must be old enough to have decades of medical expe-

rience, yet young enough to be in touch with next year's technology. Must have an outstanding staff, which is voluntarily underpaid, making it possible to offer the most up-to-date service at minimal cost. Will schedule appointments for unlimited amounts of time with each patient to whom he or she devotes undivided attention. Must never require anyone to wait. Will return phone calls within five minutes while adhering to a full surgical schedule to keep skills sharp. Must work long hours, yet intelligently discuss the plot of last night's sitcoms to put patients at ease. Must have the humility to say, "I don't know," or "I need help," but will never need to say either. Will instantly be able to assess whether a patient needs a strong dose of hope or caution. Must never say the wrong thing. Is a genius, yet sociable, sensitive and, witty. Must have a reputation for demonstrating a wonderful bedside manner. Is always in a good mood, and can handle with ease and pleasure any number of patients lacking any or all of these qualities.

Even people with lower expectations than I have usually struggled to keep the doctor/patient relationship in perspective. After all, our schedules, our checkbooks, and our hopes begin to revolve around them. We recall every word they say, replaying conversations endlessly.

Meanwhile, our medical practitioners often seem incapable of remembering our names, not to mention previous conversations, diagnoses, surgeries, even miscarriages.

What's a patient to do?

We start by working with the right physician.

Choosing a Physician

"Choosing a doctor for your infertility workup is like shopping for a coat," writes patient Jody Earle. "Some you don't like; some you can't afford; some don't meet your needs. Some look great on someone else; some don't fit. Eventually, you find one which will feel comfortable and seem just right for you. . . .

"Above all else, remember that you, the consumer, have to be pleased with your purchase. If you're not, change it, because you're not likely to use a purchase which you don't like."[1]

But how do you start looking? Titles such as reproductive endocrinologist, gynecologist, and infertility specialist can be so confusing. What do they mean? Dr. Bill explains:

After graduating from college, a student attends four years of medical school to receive an M.D. degree and the title of physician. To specialize in obstetrics/gynecology, the new physician then completes a four-year program with relatively little emphasis on infertility. However, having completed this, Ob/Gyns can call themselves "infertility specialists"—or even "God"—if they want to. Urologists take three years to complete specialty training, in an "earn as you learn" program that likewise limits exposure to infertility. This is simply because "common problems are common," and instructors focus most of their students' training on the "dramatically affected" hospital patient. Exposure to office evaluation of the infertile couple is minimal.

To demonstrate proficiency as an expert, the doctor must immediately take a written examination. After two years' practice he is eligible to take an oral board examination, which may not even address infertility issues. After passing these, he or she becomes a board-certified obstetrics/gynecology specialist. These physicians often skillfully perform medium- and low-tech procedures such as Clomid therapy, inseminations, and diagnostic and operative laparoscopy. All Ob/Gyns receive some infertility training in their residencies. Most can do basic evaluations, which will often uncover problems treatable with standard therapy. The question of when to refer patients for more complex therapies is a judgment call. As one director of a Texas IVF clinic says, "I see a lot of referrals from doctors who have started evaluations, and though there are always times when I'd like to have seen them handle a case differently, most have done a good job."

Specialists agree that some Ob/Gyns understand and can evaluate infertility well while others cannot. And most Ob/Gyns know little to nothing of male infertility. The general rule is that if you have been with a physician six to twelve months and have no diagnosis nor a pregnancy, it seems reasonable to pursue another option.

Women generally consult their Ob/Gyns first. Some couples find it difficult to continue seeing an obstetrician for infertility because they would rather avoid pregnant women. Seeing enlarged stomachs and baby magazines in the waiting area can hurt, and they may even have to reschedule appointments because the doctor is out delivering babies. On the other hand, some women prefer to stay with an obstetrician for fertility treatment because they want continuity of care should conception occur. Geography may also limit the number of specialists available.

To subspecialize, the gynecologist completes a two-year fellowship in reproductive endocrinology and infertility. After an additional year of research and after publishing a thesis in a fertility medical journal, the sub-specialist becomes board-eligible in the field of infertility. Once again, he or she must take a written and an oral examination to become a board-certified subspecialist in the field of reproductive endocrinology and infertility. Generally, these are the physicians you see in charge of high-tech programs such as *in vitro* clinics. Many of these highly specialized physicians will not even see patients unless Ob/Gyns have already performed initial evaluations.

Most of the high-tech practices offer the advantages of seven-day-a-week staff availability, transvaginal ultrasound equipment, and on-site certified labs.

Contact on-line support groups, a RESOLVE chapter, (RESOLVE offers physician referral to members) or other patients for physician recommendations. Then choose a physician whose educational training and approach fit your desires, whether conservative or aggressive. Base your decision on his or her ability to perform the procedures you want or need, keeping in mind that generally a higher level of training and availability translate into a higher price tag.

Some questions to ask might include the following: Is she a reproductive endocrinologist? Does he have special training or interest in infertility? Where did the medical team get their training? Can you ask other patients about accessibility, sensitivity, and communication skills?

The Gender Question

What about gender differences in choosing a doctor? Some Christians insist that wives see only female doctors and husbands go only to males. I strongly disagree. Either gender can provide quality medical care without violating the person of the patient. I have heard about and read of physicians taking advantage of patients, but most have high standards of personal ethics and deserve patients' trust. It is far more critical to have a caring, competent physician who can communicate than to focus on gender.

It might help at this point to reveal a well-kept secret—what goes on (or rather, what doesn't) in the physician's mind during the infertility investigation. First, about the examination: The female anatomy is fairly standardized so that no one is so "remarkable" as to be "memorable."

Then there's the ongoing treatment. Most patients think I remember when they're supposed to have sex or the phase of the cycle in which they find themselves. Sorry. My mind is full enough, as I suspect is true for most practitioners, without retaining details, fantasies, or even judgmental thoughts. I cannot keep most facts, tests, temperatures, and family situations in my memory. That's why we use charts. Certainly, after months of testing I try to get to know and understand individual couples better, but still, the many details recorded in the office chart remain there.

I cannot count the times I've run into patients at football games or at the mall, and they have asked me detailed questions. I simply don't know the answers without the facts in front of me. I'm pretty good with names, so I can usually exchange a greeting. But most prefer their privacy. For this reason, I generally avoid initiating conversation. I steer away from raising questions among their friends which they would rather not have to answer.

My mind is so compartmentalized that before entering a patient's exam room, I review the chart to see where we've been and where we're going. Then I open the door and fix my full attention on that one patient. Ideally, I can focus so there is "no other patient in the world" for the duration of the visit. This way I can ask all the necessary questions with total concentration. I make notes on the chart to trigger my thinking for future visits. When I leave the room, I begin to focus on the next medical need. If there is an important date for testing or results, I indicate it in my notes. For the time allotted, that patient is the center of my attention.

Some patients have expressed embarrassment when coming in immediately after sex for a "post coital test." They wonder if I've looked at my watch and thought about what they were doing. I certainly never envision wine, music, and bodies entwined. I don't violate their privacy as much as they might think. If anything, upon seeing a post coital test on the schedule, my only thoughts are hopes that they succeed. I've had hundreds of calls over the years from couples who just couldn't "perform" under pressure.

Oprah Winfrey asked several male gynecologists on her show, "Do sexual thoughts ever enter your mind during the exam?"

One said, "No. It's no different from examining a knee or an ear."

Another explained, "There are no sexual thoughts. I am working very hard to make the patient feel as comfortable as possible; that takes a lot of effort and confidence and energy. We want to get the exam over as quickly as we can. Basically, when a patient is in a gown and a sheet, there's no sexual connotation. I am doing my job."

A female gynecologist recommends that rather than making gender an issue, "Select your physician for compassion, availability, competence, and communication."

Working with Your Physician

Two weeks after a head-on collision, I [Sandi] sat with my friend, Gina, in her hospital room. The driver who caused the wreck had died. Gina had a compound fracture in her right leg, and the four pins piercing her flesh pushed the limits of what I could stomach.

The physical therapist breezed in, woke her abruptly, and declared, "The doctor wants you to take a few steps today."

Gina gazed at me as if to plead, "Don't let her do this to me." We were both appalled at the suggestion. Gina couldn't even sit up in a wheelchair without passing out.

Don't question her doctor's judgment, I reminded myself. *Surely he knows what he's doing.* I clamped my tongue with my teeth. The therapist sat her up, though Gina begged to lay back down. When her mangled leg touched the floor, she screamed and collapsed on the bed. Feeling myself start to pass out, I groped for the nearest chair. The therapist looked at me helplessly and said softly, "I'm just trying to do what the doctor said."

Someone had made a mistake. When Gina's new therapist arrived the next day, he gave her some advice: "Your doctor or therapist may tell you what to do, but neither of them is ultimately in charge of your treatment. You are in charge. Don't be helpless. Work together with them. If you know you're trying your hardest and they demand more, you don't have to do it. Only you really know your limits. You have to control the situation instead of letting it control you. You're the manager. Remember, you're paying *us* to serve *you.*"

That accident happened when I was in the early stages of infertility treatment. (Today, only a few small scars remind Gina of her ordeal.) Later, as I read 1 Corinthians 6:19–20, the words took on new meaning: " Do you know that your body is a temple of the Holy Spirit who is in you, whom you have from God, and that you are not your own? For you have been bought with a price: therefore glorify God in your body." I realized that I alone would give account for what I'd done, actively or passively, with my body—that God held me ultimately responsible. As a result, I began to manage my own medical care, reading extensively, writing questions, and expecting teamwork.

According to a *Consumer Reports* survey of seventy thousand people, most people feel satisfied with their doctors care, but half are unhappy with at least one aspect of their treatment, particularly communication. One in four said their doctors did not warn of possible side effects from medication, and one in five complained that their physicians failed to encourage questions. People whose physicians didn't communicate well with them were less likely to follow instructions.[2]

Other research indicates that satisfied patients comply more fully with instructions. Another study conducted among severely burned children showed that those who changed and dressed their own burns required less medication. They also experienced fewer complications than patients who did not. Researchers concluded that taking an active role in medical treatment promotes healing.

Still other studies show that patients who ask questions and expect answers experience less physical discomfort, have more positive attitudes, and feel more in control than passive patients. As a result, they suffer from less stress and are better able to deal with their problems.

Often patients blame their doctors for poor communication, but Chicago researchers found that, especially when the news is bad, many patients don't process the information as intended. Apparently, survival instincts set in, making it hard for patients to hear what their physicians are really saying.

So how can we do our part to promote better doctor/patient relationships? Here are some suggestions:

- Before having any test done, have your doctor explain its cost, purpose, average success rate, and expected outcome. Ask if he or she has a written information sheet—or knows where you can get one—about the procedure.
- Write down your questions ahead of time. Periodically schedule appointments separate from tests and examinations during which you discuss only test results and treatment plans. Many patients complain that their brains turn to Jell-O as soon as they're dressed in surgical gowns, feeling that their ability to think is inversely related to the size

of the slit up the back. Allow yourself to hold some discussions in nonthreatening circumstances.

- Bring your spouse as often as possible. Most couples who go together can recount times when one heard information the other did not catch. Together you can do a better job of piecing together the treatment puzzle.

- If you need it, take extra time to make decisions. Avoid rushing. This is your body and your money. If your mind goes blank during the consultation and you agree to follow a plan you're uncomfortable with later, resolve difficulties before moving ahead. Don't feel "locked in" to doing something you're unsure about.

- Refrain from taking any medications unless you understand why you're taking them. Be sure you understand how to take them, and know the possible side effects.

- Don't expect your physician to be an expert in areas outside of his or her expertise. Most doctors do not hold degrees in counseling and psychology. If you want emotional support, talk to a friend, a pastor, or a therapist.

- As indicated earlier, expect that your doctor will remember few details of your life and treatment without your file handy. Although these seem impossible for you to forget, even the most caring physician rarely focuses a lot of thought on individual patients once they have left his or her office. After a year of constant visits to one clinic, the staff still thought my husband's name was Richard instead of Gary; and the physician kept forgetting I'd ever had a miscarriage. Yes, I felt annoyed, but I also received excellent medical care. I knew they felt genuine concern for me, even if they failed to remember the most important person in my life.

- Cultivate good relationships with the support staff. As most ongoing contact is with the staff rather than the physician, work hard at building rapport with the nurses and clerical team. A skilled nursing staff consulting with the physician can manage most questions. Many patients want to speak only to the doctor, which often brings unnecessary delays. The physician should be aware of test results, progress, and decisions in each case, but he should not necessarily be the only person who can communicate them.

- Call before you leave the house or job to see if the doctor is running late. This can help you avoid long delays in the waiting room. Also, plan to take a book or project with you so you won't have to reread that same issue of *People* twenty-five times.

- Get clarification when necessary. *Feel free to call the office and ask questions.* When you get test results, ask for normal values. Repeat the doctor's or nurse's instructions so you're sure you've understood correctly.

When the Medical Team Fails

Notice we didn't say "if" they fail, we said "when." If you're going to the doctor's office and awaiting blood test results several times a week, month after month, sooner or later you'll encounter misunderstandings, delays, and even major mistakes. I have to laugh now when I read through my journal. On one day I was so frustrated with one of my doctors that I called him a "turkey" and "slug bait" all day. (Not to his face, of course.)

"Do we expect too much in asking doctors to speak English and not only 'Hysterosalpingogram'? asks Dan Clements, former chair of RESOLVE, Inc. "Is it too much to ask the doctor to understand that our mere presence in their office is upsetting, and we need time to digest their words and formulate our questions? And that our questions do not imply a lack of trust, but rather are evidence of an insatiable need to understand the facts so we can participate in the decisions? We, as patients, must remember that we are not the doctor's only patient and not the only blocked tube in town. It is our responsibility to educate ourselves as much as possible outside the doctor's office as well as inside. It would be nice, however, if all doctors understood that our blocked tubes may not be the only ones in town, but they are our only set, and their blockage is breaking our hearts."

Allison, a fertility patient in Georgia, tells about her gyne-cologist who prescribed drugs for discomfort. Upon chang-ing doctors, Allison learned that the medication had effectively worked as birth control for a year. "Not only had I wasted a year of potential fertility," she writes, "I had diffi-culty with my emotional response to the medication, and I have recently learned that it put me in a higher risk group for cancer. I'm still a little angry. My doctor should have done more research; I should have done more research. Doctors are people, patients are people, and people can only do the best they can do at a given time. I have to forgive her and myself. Allowing myself to accept the imperfections of humans does make me feel better."

Once, a doctor put me on complete bed rest because Per-gonal had hyperstimulated my ovaries—a potentially dan-gerous condition. I went into his office for a sonogram, which the nurse performed. As I was leaving, he walked through the office and noticed my eyes clouding over. He reassured me with, "I'm going to call you today."

Two days later, I still lay in bed awaiting his call. Finally, I picked up the phone and waded through the multileveled screening structure, demanding to talk to him. He humbly admitted that I could have been at work for the past two days because the sonogram results had shown that I was fine. He had forgotten to call me because someone had refiled my chart, effectively removing his reminder. "I knew I'd forgotten something when I went to bed last night," he told me, "but I just couldn't remember what it was." Fortu-nately, my anger had finally driven me to call, and I let him know his neglect hurt.

Why didn't I change doctors? Because I knew patients who saw all the other major infertility doctors in my city and in many other states. I knew I encountered fewer of these problems than most of them did. Some difficulties are inevitable. I had to remind myself that God was in control even when my doctor made mistakes.

Infertility investigations are complex and can span many months. Eventually some test results will be delayed or not reported quickly. The staff tries hard to prevent anyone from "slipping through the cracks," but physicians who have seen no test results are thinking about the patients currently in the office. Thus, when a delay occurs, the patient will usually realize it before the physician will.

I [Bill] try to explain when to expect test results so that if they don't come in, we will either catch it or the patient will know when to call. We are happy for patients to call about test results. This is where a good working relationship with the office team can be a blessing. If the patients call us, they don't sit around the house fuming because we haven't called; otherwise, the office staff busily works away oblivious to the gathering storm.

We make mistakes. Tests may be scheduled incorrectly. Doctors called at home—away from vital information—may give inadequate advice. Even the best physician, despite what he or she may think, is fallible. In fact, contrary to what one company claims ("We make babies"), we know that God alone makes babies. We do what we can to improve the environment, enhancing the possibilities based on the technology God has permitted us to use. But conception, the alignment and functioning of chromosomes, happens independently of our medical manipulation.

When problems arise or mistakes happen, I firmly believe the patient should approach the physician and communicate the circumstances. Biblically, he or she should resolve any differences, seeking wise counsel from trained spiritual individuals, if necessary. Whether or not the physician is a believer, the believing patient must act in a Christlike manner, speaking up about what is wrong, while demonstrating grace and forgiveness. When the physician is the one who recognizes the mistake, I believe he or she must initiate disclosure and reconciliation. Do not hesitate to call your physician's office if something unusual happens! Most physicians deeply desire to do what is right and best, and accurate information from educated, involved patients helps immeasurably.

Get the best care you can find. Participate actively in your treatment; work hard at "giving away grace" when someone messes up. If at the end of it all you still have no children, you will be able to assure yourself that you did all you could to get the best help modern science had to offer, and you retained your dignity in the process.

One Saturday as Gary and I [Sandi] sat in a waiting room, we overheard a patient blowing a gasket because the doctor planned to go out of town to attend a fertility society's annual meeting. It meant she would have to see his partner.

"How dare you plan a trip which fails to accommodate all your patients' cycles," we joked with him later. He just shook his head and sighed.

WANTED: Patients with realistic expectations.

How fitting the reminder, "My soul, wait thou only upon God; for my expectation is from him (Ps. 62:5, KJV).

For Further Reading

Rank, Maureen. *Free to Grieve.* Minneapolis, Minn.: Bethany House, 1985. Excellent chapter on "When the Medical Team Fails."

Robin, Peggy. *How to Be a Successful Fertility Patient: Your Guide to Getting the Best Possible Medical Help to Have a Baby.* New York, N.Y.: William Morrow & Co, 1993. This guide is a great resource for consumers of fertility health-care services.

For Couples' Discussion

1. Are you getting the best medical care possible?
2. Are you taking seriously your responsibility to manage your own care?
3. What do you expect from your physician/staff team?
4. Are your expectations realistic?
5. Do you need to expect more or less from them?
6. Are you expecting the medical team to have expert knowledge in areas in which they are untrained?
7. Have you experienced "slipups" with the doctor or office staff? If so, do you need to speak up? Do you need to "let it go"?
8. Read 2 Chronicles 16:11–12. In whom are you trusting?

He that is slow to anger is better than the mighty;
And he that ruleth his spirit than he that taketh a city.

—*Proverbs 16:32, KJV*

Chapter 7

What Do We Do
with Our Anger?

"Watch out for stray lightning bolts," I wrote across the top of the page. I'd found a letter an infertility patient had written to God, and it sizzled with anger. Dr. Bill was putting together a lecture on the spiritual and emotional effects of infertility, and I was gathering some information for him when I found it. Here's a shortened version of the letter:

Dear God,

As you most certainly know by now, I don't have any faith whatsoever in you. I don't even like you. I think you've done a lousy job of supervising the frail planet on which I live. Under normal circumstances, you'd be fired. You must have terrific tenure.

Nonetheless, I couldn't find anybody else old enough and big enough to talk to. I've noticed a lot of other humans whispering to you, mumbling their thanks, quietly requesting everything from profit-sharing to eternal salvation. I'm not asking for anything. I just want to let you know that I'm angry. Filled with rage that's got twenty thousand years of savage mating behind it. And I want to explode it at your heaven.

I cannot have children. Like Abraham's wife, Sarah. Remember her? A barren womb, empty arms. Of all the plagues and curses and disasters you have sent to earth, this is the most wicked. It is incomprehensible.

Nothing you schemed was quite as treacherous as the human heart. You connected it to everything. Every sight and every gesture, every cell in every tissue in every organ in every body registers somewhere in the heart. To touch a new baby, to contemplate eternity, to ovulate, to bury a grandmother, to love a man—these, and a thousand other events coagulate, and somewhere in the thick purple muscle of the heart, form a longing: to have children. It is not an irrational desire. It is, in fact, the natural order of things. It is unnatural only inside a woman who is barren. Then this longing, this sweet harmless longing, turns on itself, clogs the openings to the heart, spreads over the entire surface of the heart, hardening many of the tender spots, breaking it in places, and finally, in desperation, exploding. All that is left is a great gaping hole that will never be filled.

You ask more than is reasonable.

Amen.[1]

I called Dr. Bill after I'd sent him the stack of materials. "Did you see my note about the lightning bolt?" I asked him.
"Yes."
"What did you think of that letter?"
"I guess I had a different response. I saw it as an honest expression of pain, which God welcomes. He's big enough to handle it. Sometimes when we discover God gives us the freedom to misunderstand Him, we can arrive at an even greater love and respect for Him."

I reread my copy and wept. *Is He not outraged?* I asked myself. I wasn't sure.

Several years and miscarriages later, we began working with a teenaged birth mother, Renee, who wanted us to adopt her unborn daughter. As one who had been abused as a child, Renee confided in me that she had slugged the baby *in utero* when it kicked too hard. Naturally, we were concerned. I went with her to see the ultrasound. She said she wanted me to be there for the labor and delivery. So, for the first time in years, I endured hanging out with pregnant women, telling myself, "It's worth it—in the end we'll have a baby," and I went with her to birthing classes, acting as her coach.

A call came that another little girl had been born. Did we want to adopt immediately? We said no, because Renee was due in less than a month. She was depending on us. So another friend adopted that child.

Then Renee's call came. Two weeks before her due date, she decided to keep the baby. We felt devastated. What about that poor child who had already suffered abuse? Nevertheless, we had peace that we'd made the right decisions.

Amazingly, another birth mother called that week. She was due in another month. She asked if we would fly her in to stay with us for a weekend so she could feel good about the family that might be adopting her child. We felt emotionally spent, but we decided we'd better take the opportunity. So we did. We really liked Marcy. She was a Christian who wanted to place her child in a believing home. We prayed together and spent hours by the fire talking.

While she was with us, we received a call that one of my husband's closest friends had died suddenly of complications from diabetes. As we sat at his funeral, we learned that Renee was in labor. I thought, *We were supposed to become parents today, and instead all we have is multiple losses.*

We continued to focus on Marcy's baby and began to get the nursery ready. Then, three days before Christmas, we called. When we reached her, we learned that she had given birth to a little girl that morning, and she had decided to keep the baby. I couldn't believe that the God I love and serve had allowed this to happen.

My sister called and said, "You're playing 'The Wheel of Misfortune,' aren't you? Why don't you fly to California and go skiing with us? In two months you've lost three opportunities to have a child. Come on. We can go to Lake Tahoe." So we booked a flight.

I flung myself across the bed and prayed, "Lord, have mercy! Let something go right." I'm sorry to say that it was the first time I'd talked to Him in three days.

When we got to California, my niece got chicken pox. Lake Tahoe was full, so we had to choose another place to ski. The condominium we had booked didn't have a private bedroom for us, as we had been told it would. So my husband and I had to try to talk through our grief in the middle of the living room with small children interrupting. Everything seemed to continue in a downward spiral. Again, I flung myself across the bed and cried to the Lord, "Have *mercy!*"

Weeks earlier I had agreed to write a Bible study on the Psalms for the women in my church. So I sent everyone to the slopes the following morning. I told them, "I'll feel less pressure if I can get something written. Give me a few hours to myself."

The first Psalm I had chosen was Psalm 22. It begins, "My God, my God, why have you forsaken me?" I had always heard this psalm in the context of Jesus on the cross, but I had never seen that it had been originally written by David, out of his own experience. For the first time I saw from the Scriptures themselves that God allows, even invites, our expressions of negative feelings. Certainly God had not forsaken David, but David *felt* like He had. David had accused God of hitting the road, and, amazingly, God included his complaint in Scripture for our benefit.

As I studied, I began to find more and more such expressions. In *Cry of the Soul,* Dan Allender observes this phenomenon:

> The psalmist brings his struggle to God and, at times, accuses Him of being faithless—even a lousy businessman. "You gave us up to be devoured like sheep and have scattered us among the nations," he scolds God. "You sold your people for a pittance, gaining nothing from their sale" (44:11–12). He wags his

finger at God's face, accusing Him not only of negligence, but idiocy.

Elsewhere the psalmist furiously mocks God for bringing pain into his life:

You have taken from me my closest friends

and have made me repulsive to them.

I am confined and cannot escape;

my eyes are dim with grief.

I call to you, O LORD, every day

I spread out my hands to you. (88:8–9, NIV)

Allender goes on to observe, "Some believers cringe from this language of desperation and rage, even though they have the model of the psalmist. . . . The Psalms invite us to question God, but they do this in the context of worship—they were the hymnal used in public worship. God invites us to bring before Him our rage, doubt, and terror—but He intends for us to do so as part of worship. This is the kind of emotional struggle we must engage in if we are to fathom the nature of God's heart for us."[2]

In his work titled *Prayer: Finding the Heart's True Home,* Richard Foster writes, "Lament [psalms] often express anger, accusations against enemies, and criticism of God for not taking action or answering prayers. We may want to reject such psalms with their negative words, but we may also admit that sometimes we feel the same feelings they convey. Laments express honesty, realism, and integrity. They keep the conversation with God open and help break down our isolation in times of suffering. God encourages us to keep talking even when our thinking is mixed up with negative thoughts and we say things we ordinarily would not. Laments give us permission to shake our fist at God one minute and break into songs of praise the next."[3]

So anger isn't wrong? Considering that the Bible includes nearly four hundred specific references to anger, most of which refer to the anger of God, we can conclude that anger by itself is not an evil emotion.

"I have become confident that most persons are, at best, thoroughly confused about anger," writes Neil Warren, Ph.D., in *Make Anger Your Ally*. "They are unaware of any difference between anger and aggression; they have almost never distinguished between anger and hostility. Anger remains for them a largely unexplored subject which causes frustration and feelings of hopelessness."[4]

I saw the invitation in the Psalms to express my anger (which ranges from frustration to rage) to God in the context of worship. Still I felt reluctant to do so. I wondered if other Scriptures carried this same invitation, so I did some research.

First I found this from Jeremiah, "the weeping prophet": "O LORD, you deceived me, and I was deceived; you overpowered me and prevailed. I am ridiculed all day long, everyone mocks me. Whenever I speak, I cry out proclaiming violence and destruction.

So the word of the LORD has brought me insult and reproach all day long" (Jer. 20:7–8, NIV).

He accused God of deception? Really? I read on.

"How long, O LORD, must I call for help, but you do not listen? Or cry out to you, 'Violence!' but you do not save?" (Hab. 1:2–4, NIV).

Habakkuk also felt free to complain about God's slowness to answer. Then I looked at Gideon, who asked, "If the Lord is with us, why has all this happened to us?" Again, God didn't rebuke him; He reassured him.

Job initially fell on his face and worshiped; but when his emotional and physical pain went on and on, he began to question God. Jonah got upset because he didn't like God showing mercy to His enemies. He sulked, then he became angry. (The word *anger* occurs six times in the final chapter.) Here again, God patiently worked with His quarreling servant.

Moses argued. Peter disagreed. Then I found Mary, Martha's sister, who expressed unhappiness about Jesus' absence: "Lord, if you had been here, this wouldn't have happened." Jesus didn't rebuke her; He wept at Lazarus' tomb. Even the Book of Revelation quotes martyred saints living in heaven (thus sinless) wondering, "How long, O Lord, holy and true, will you refrain from judging and avenging our blood?" These people were in a perfected state asking God questions!

This began to make more sense to me when I took my kitten, Jellico, to the veterinarian for shots. As I drove, he grew terrified. He wouldn't sit still or let me hold him. He cried and climbed all over the interior of my car. Because I operate on a different level of intelligence than Jellico does, I had no way of explaining to him on his level that I had his best interest at heart. He knew only fear. I would not have become angry with him if he had hissed at me. I would have known he was only expressing logical emotions. Based on the Scriptures, I have to believe God feels the same way about us.

Instead of viewing my relationship with God as merely master/servant, I began to see it more like a partnership or friendship. Servants generally don't express opinions, but spouses question and express frustration. Jesus called the disciples His friends; Paul calls the church the "bride of Christ."

In the process of observing this invitation to express emotion to God, I found that many of these expressions occurred in the context of prayer. Most of us would rather make our complaints public, but we never take the time to pray. God encourages us to come directly to Him with our beefs. I am not suggesting that we conjure up anger toward God; but at some point, everyone will probably wrestle with these feelings. When we do, we have the assurance that struggling people fill the Scriptures. We can tell our loving Heavenly Father that we're upset, and find rest in Him.

So it's all right to be angry at God? Is it all right for a child to be unhappy with his parents when things aren't going his way? Of course. As we watch those of our friends who are loving, yet imperfect, earthly parents, we see them encouraging their children to express their feelings. Our perfectly loving Heavenly Father desires our presence even if it means pouring out our hearts in anger, frustration, and fear. Only here can God minister to the deep needs of our hearts and teach the deep truths of immovable, unshakable faith. At times, God's seeming distance and apparent silence work to draw us nearer in silence so we can appreciate His love, sense His voice, and feel His tender touch on our lives.

We often have the wrong idea about anger. We think "truly spiritual people feel only positive emotions," but it's not immature to feel angry; it's immature to stay angry.

I heard a professor share with a group of students that when he and his wife first married they experienced conflict, like any couple. He confessed that sometimes days passed before they spoke to each other again, but their love matured through time.

Years later, he rushed around getting ready for a trip, exasperated because a thousand little details had gone wrong; and he let his wife know it. But as he reached for the door knob, he stopped. Then he turned around, looked at her, and said, "Baby, I'm sorry." She ran and threw her arms around him. "Honey," she exclaimed, "you've got it down to fifteen seconds!"

Now, that's maturity. Being mature as a Christian doesn't mean we're never upset. It means developing the habit of moving more quickly from lament to praise. During most of my infertility experience, I thought the one place I could not express my anger was in God's presence. Now I know that the one truly legitimate place to take it is to Him.

One patient, Robyn, shares,

> A friend called and asked me to join her and some friends for a make-over session. Feeling this might boost my confidence a little, I agreed. Five other women came that evening to her house. Two had babies with them. One was pregnant and due any day. We had just about wrapped it up for the evening, when one of the women announced she was pregnant. Everyone exclaimed for joy. Then the other woman announced that she, too, was pregnant.

> Heading back, the freeway turned into a blur in front of me. I realized that my evening hadn't exactly turned out the way I had planned. I had a talk with God. I was

glad I was alone. I wanted to be honest and let out what I was *really* feeling, pretty or not—not the way I thought this perfect Christian woman should be reacting but how I was actually feeling.

"Why do I feel like you are punishing me?" I cried out. "When is the suffering and the heartache going to end? Why me? I don't understand." Then, after the tears slowed and I paused in silence, I decided that no matter what God brought into my life, no matter how much suffering I felt I would have to endure with this emptiness in my heart longing for a baby, I would never stop loving Him.

So how do we get from point A (anger) to point B (praise)? The Psalms provide wonderful examples of how to express ourselves.

"I went down to the land
  whose bars closed upon me forever;
  yet you brought up my life from the Pit,
  O LORD my God.
  As my life was ebbing away,

I remembered the LORD;
  and my prayer came to you,
  into your holy temple.
  Those who worship vain idols
  forsake their true loyalty.

But I with my voice of thanksgiving
  will sacrifice to you;
  what I have vowed I will pay.
  Deliverance belongs to the LORD!"

Jonah 2:6–9, authors' paraphrase

Actually, this is part of Jonah's prayer as he lies in the belly of the fish. But it looks like it's from the Psalms, doesn't it?

In his marvelous work on Jonah, *Under the Unpredictable Plant,* Eugene Peterson writes:

Not one word in [Jonah's] prayer is original. Jonah got every word—lock, stock and barrel—out of his Psalms book. . . . The commonest form of prayer in the

Psalms is the lament. It is what we would expect, since it is our commonest condition. We are in trouble a lot, so we pray in the lament form a lot. A graduate of the Psalms School of Prayer would like this form best of all, by sheer force of repetition. . . . Circumstances dictated "lament." But prayer, while influenced by circumstances, is not determined by them. Jonah, creative in his praying, chose to pray in the form of "praise."

If we want to pray our true condition, our total selves in response to the living God, expressing our feelings is not enough—we need a long apprenticeship in prayer. And then we need graduate school. The Psalms are the school. . . . Prayer rescues us from a preoccupation with ourselves and pulls us into adoration of and pilgrimage to God.[5]

We need to let our emotions take us to the Psalms, where we pray the time-tested prayers that move us from lament to praise.

"Why, Lord?"

"How long, O Lord?"

"Do you love me?"

God invites us to ask these legitimate questions. He could make us fertile if He wanted to, but He chooses not to, and *that* upsets us.

So why isn't He doing anything? Or is He?

Suggested Reading

Allender, Dan, Ph.D, M.Div. and Tremper Longman, Ph.D., M.Div. *Cry of the Soul: How our Emotions Reveal our Deepest Questions About God.* Colorado Springs, Colo.: NavPress, 1994, 36–37.

The Book of Psalms.

For Couples' Discussion

1. What do you usually do with your negative feelings?
2. Do you feel free to express them to God?
3. Read Psalm 88 and Lamentations 3. Do you identify with the emotions expressed?
4. Spend some time talking to God about your frustrations.

Chapter 8

Am I Infertile
Because I Did Something Wrong?

Susie skipped church one Wednesday evening to help decorate the float her high school class was building for a parade. Even though she was only fifteen, she had her driver's license and had obtained permission to borrow her father's truck. When she arrived at the deserted hangar her group used for their traditional decorating activities, no one was there. The time and place had changed, but her classmates had forgotten to tell her. As Susie was leaving the airport, the driver in the car behind her kept flashing his lights. So she pulled over and rolled down her window just a crack.

"Your truck's on fire!" the man told her, "but don't worry. I'll help you." She knew the closest help was several miles down the road, but not wanting to trust a stranger, she took off for the gas station. The other driver followed, continuing to flash his lights. Finally Susie pulled over in a residential area and got out of the truck. She thought she smelled fire and rubber burning, but she didn't see any flames.

"I'll take you," he said. Then he grabbed her and threw her back into the truck. She hit the door on other side and grabbed the lock, which broke off in her hand. She began banging against the door screaming, "Help me!"

"You'd better shut up or I'll put this through you," he growled, motioning to a knife. Susie sat frozen with fear as he drove them out of town to the city dump.

Susie's abductor raped and stabbed her multiple times. Then he unrolled twine from samples that her father, a carpet salesman, had left in the back of his truck. He wrapped it around her neck in an effort to choke her. After that, he buried her in the garbage and stole her vehicle.

Susie managed to stand up and search for the city lights. She headed toward them, eventually walking about three miles. As she moved, she could hear air expiring from the stab wounds to her lungs. She sat down to rest once, but she could feel life slipping away. So she pushed herself on. When she finally found the highway, she waved down a man who picked her up and put her in the bed of his truck because his cab was full. He took her to the closest truck stop.

In the meantime, Susie's abductor had wrecked her father's truck and the wreckage had sent her father and the police looking for her sometime close to midnight. Susie arrived at the truck stop only seconds before her dad and the police pulled up. "They came to the bed of the truck to I.D. me," she remembers, "and my Dad told them, 'Yes, she's my daughter; my baby girl.'"

A few moments later, an ambulance arrived; within several hours police arrested the rapist at his home. He had stabbed Susie three times in the abdomen, so she had to be rushed to major surgery. Afterwards, nurses tried to wash her hair, which was caked with blood and muck from the dump. She had broken blood vessels in her face, so her mother kept mirrors away from her.

Susie had just become a believer that summer. Her friends, relatives, and church family held prayer vigils. She knew God had not caused her assaulter to attack, but she had thoughts such as, "If only I'd gone to church that night, this wouldn't have happened." Through this experience

Susie's grandparents came to know Christ, but she wondered, "Why did it have to be so drastic?"

Years later, when Susie married, she and her husband began trying to have a baby. Before long, they realized something was wrong. Then came even more horror. An armed serial rapist hid in Susie's garage, and she experienced rape a second time. She cried out to God saying, "This is unfair. Why didn't You protect me? I know You didn't do it. But You allowed it to happen!"

I [Bill] remember vividly the phone call as Susie shared this terrible event with me. After covering the necessary medical issues, I tried to comfort and encourage her. I could barely speak as my heart broke for her. How unbelievably, incredibly unfair! Could anyone withstand such psychological pressure? I doubt my words were any comfort, but I wanted to reach out and make this go away. I wanted to minister to this family's need and to somehow solve the fertility puzzle, that their weeping might be replaced with joy.

This time Susie knew of no one who benefited from her pain. "For awhile I felt like I'd kill myself if it happened again," she remembers. "My husband wasn't pushy about sexual intimacy. If he wanted to make advances and I'd say, 'Don't touch me,' he was very patient. He sought counsel from our pastor, which helped."

Susie went to counseling this time, but her therapist was no help—he told her she should consider it a "compliment" to be raped. So she quit seeing him. She suppressed her emotions for a long time.

I thought their fertility problem might be caused by a low-grade infection from the rape or the adhesions from exploratory surgery. So I performed a laparoscopy, which indeed demonstrated tubal damage, possibly resulting from disease secondary to the rapes, surgery complications, or both. I had more bad news for Susie. *Where is this "wise benevolence" from our sovereign God?* I wondered.

I recommended laparotomy and attempted to microsurgically repair the tubal damage. I quoted the less-than-optimistic percentages for success. Susie remembers, "The surgery fixed the problem, but we discovered others along the way. Each time a new problem arose, my faith would get very shaky. I would cry out, 'Why can't I have this baby I want so badly?' I have always loved babies. It had never occurred to me that my desire might be an impossibility."

Then she had good news. She was finally pregnant. I remember the day. I don't know how physicians can remain "distant and not personally involved." What joy to be a part of this pregnancy! Susie's dream of having a baby came true with a healthy boy.

"Life was great," she says, thinking back on that time. "I thought, *God works things out.* When she gave birth to a second son she was ecstatic, but after that her emotions plummeted. She found a counselor who helped her sort out her feelings, and she spent months, working through her fear, anxiety, and excruciating emotional pain.

Is Infertility a Punishment from God?

Considering how far we fall short of God's standard, we must recognize that a just and holy God would be justified if He chose to punish us. Jeremiah asked, "Why should any living mortal . . . offer complaint in view of his sins?" (Lam. 3:39).

Yet we see that God describes John the Baptist's parents, Elisabeth and Zecharias as "righteous" at the time of their infertility. Rabbi Michael Gold has observed, "Infertility in the Bible is usually not a punishment but, on the contrary, an affliction of the most pious.[1]

Nevertheless, we know that God sometimes disciplines His children. Hebrews 12:6-8 reads, "For those whom the Lord loves He disciplines. . . . for what son is there whom his father does not discipline?" Also, 1 Corinthians 11 teaches that believers in the first-century church in Corinth had become weak, sick, and were even dying because they had failed to examine themselves and turn from sin.

While we know there's not always a cause/effect relationship between sin and suffering, we may still fear that our problems have come because God feels unhappy with us. We can wonder, *Is God disciplining me?* And if so, *Why?* That can lead us to play a guessing game that goes something like this: "If I can figure out what I'm doing that God doesn't like, I'll stop doing it so He'll let me have a baby."

One patient tells of her encounter with a couple who told her she needed to repent:

> We got plenty of the usual advice. But the "words of wisdom" that bothered me most came from a Christian couple who took me aside and tried to convince me that because we had taken birth control pills for four years, God was punishing us. They said that if we would only repent, we would conceive. I cried all the way home. When I told my husband what they'd said, he thought it was the silliest thing he had ever heard. He made me feel better, but the seed of doubt had been planted. Was God punishing us? Was there some unrepented sin in our lives that was causing God to discipline us? At that point and during the next few months, I scoured the Scriptures for some kind of revelation about infertility. It didn't seem to me that God punished most of the infertile women. In fact, the opposite seemed true. In most cases he had great plans for them. Sarah, Rachel, Hannah, and Elisabeth—these were righteous women who played huge roles in biblical history.

Even if we feel assured that God is not punishing us, we may still focus constantly on trying to answer "What is God trying to teach me?" Knowing our characters could always use improvement, we wonder which quality God is trying to help us develop.

We can invest a lot of negative emotional energy wondering about which of our character qualities are so underdeveloped that God would withhold a child. We may conclude, "God is delaying my ability to conceive because in my current state of character I'd be a lousy mother" (or some similar negative assessment). Of course it's possible, but one look around at all the abusive women who have given birth should reassure us that God doesn't necessarily work this way.

We often wonder what we've done wrong when bad things happen to us, or we try to guess what we're supposed to learn. That may be fine, but it's a limited perspective.

Remember the Book of Job? An innocent man endured unspeakable suffering. Then his friends came along and told him he must have done something wrong to invoke God's wrath. Actually, they started out well. For one week, they silently grieved with him; but after that, they accused him of bringing this tragedy upon himself. When Job denied their charges, they faulted him for being self-righteous.

In John's Gospel we read about a man born blind. As Jesus passed by, His disciples asked him, "Rabbi, who sinned, this man or his parents, that he should be born blind?" Jesus answered, "It was neither that this man sinned, nor his parents; but it was in order that the works of God might be displayed in him." Then Jesus healed him. The man's blindness was the vehicle through which God bestowed upon him both spiritual and physical blessing.

So we see from the Scriptures that often no cause/effect relationship exists between sin and suffering. We all sin, but not all suffering comes as result of something we have done or are doing wrong. It's always good to examine ourselves, and to confess and forsake our known sin; the Bible promises God's unconditional forgiveness. Still, those who would like to explain infertility as a sign of God's disfavor find little biblical support.

But what about the possibility that infertility is the natural consequence of wrong actions? On our last trip to the former Soviet Union, we worked with a young Christian woman who'd had an elective abortion. Infection introduced by unclean instruments used during the procedure had destroyed her tubes, leaving her with little to no chance of conceiving in the future. She told us she knew from the start that she'd made the wrong choice, and she tearfully expressed her sorrow over her actions. We shared with her verses that assured her of God's love and forgiveness. Is she living with consequences? Yes. Is God mad at her? No. Thankfully, God offers her continuing forgiveness and spiritual healing.

If we consider the physical causes of infertility, we find that most correctable sources of impaired fertility are not the result of "choices" patients make. Only abortion and sexually transmitted diseases have even the remotest causal association between infertility and behavior that violates God's guidelines. Most causes of infertility—anatomy, hormone function, sperm motility and quality, and hereditary factors—involve elements outside of the patients' control.

God has, at times, closed an individual's womb for correction, instruction, or edification. In Exodus 23:26 and Deuteronomy 7:14, God promised fertility if Israel would obey His decrees. In the "cursing" section (Deut. 28), infertility is one item on a list of national consequences. It also includes defeat in the presence of enemies, illness, boils, blindness, hemorrhoids, and mental illness to name a few. Does that mean that anytime an individual is ill or blind or has hemorrhoids, he or she is being punished by God? No. But anytime the members of the entire nation of Israel woke up and found themselves infertile, blind, sick, and depressed, they should have taken note. Nevertheless, all that has changed since the Cross (more on this in chap. 10).

Bottom line? If you're looking for a magic answer of behavior modification to make God change His mind and give you a child, you can stop searching. Confess all known sin; believe God's promises to forgive and forget; then ask Him to help you trust that He has good plans for you (even if those plans may not include children).

What Is God's Will?

We can't manipulate God by playing a guessing game of behavior modification. But does that mean we have to sit back and passively accept our circumstances as being His will? "This must be God's will for you." How many times do fertility patients hear these words from well-meaning friends? And they receive them with a variety of negative emotions.

Job didn't just "accept God's will." Nor did the man born blind. What did they do? Job cried out, railing against God. God answered with His presence and met Job's need. The man born blind asked Jesus to heal him, and He did.

Perhaps at this point it is appropriate to explain the difference between God's desired will, His allowed will, and His ultimate will.

The "desired will of God" is simply what God desires. It is for God's will to be done "on earth as it is in heaven." There would be no suffering, and everyone would live in holiness and peace, be healthy, never get sick or die, and have all their needs met. In the Garden of Eden, Adam and Eve experienced a world that fulfilled God's desired will, but God's warning to Adam was serious. Therefore, Adam's choice inaugurated a broken world full of evil and its consequences.

God's "allowed" will means He has accepted self-imposed limits, honoring the laws of human freedom and those of the universe He created. People make unwise, harmful, and even horrifying choices. From this point of view, not everything that happens is what God desires, yet He allows evil and works good through it. Thus we read in Romans 8:28 that "God causes all things to work together for good to those who love him and are called according to His purpose."

Let's look at another Bible character, Joseph. His jealous brothers sold him into slavery, and he ended up far away in Egypt. Then he was falsely accused and sat for years rotting in jail. Joseph suffered mistreatment, slander, and years of pain. Then he interpreted Pharaoh's dream and, as a result, prepared the country to endure famine. Pharaoh elevated him to a high government position. Then his brothers went to Egypt begging for food. They didn't recognize Joseph, but he knew them. He saved them from famine, and in the end he told them, "Do not be grieved or angry with yourselves, because you sold me here; for God sent me before you to preserve life. . . . And God sent me before you to preserve for you a remnant on the earth, and to keep you alive by a great deliverance. Now, therefore, it was not you who sent me here, but God; and He has made me a father to Pharaoh and lord of all his household and ruler over all the land of Egypt" (Gen. 45:5–8). We see from this story that although Joseph's brothers' actions were wrong, God allowed their evil and used it to bring about the greatest good. So even when allowing horrible circumstances, God has a loving plan.

We know that God doesn't cause sin or tempt anyone, but the lives of Job and Joseph show us that God allows suffering. Satan asked permission to strip Job of everything but life itself. God granted permission, and good came from it. Even though God restored much of what Job lost, his dead children still remained in the grave. The children God blessed Job with after his trials could not possibly replace the lives of those lost. Even though God has worked his circumstances for good (for example, we benefit from this story thousands of years later), Job still had legitimate losses to grieve. In his case, pain was not a punishment for his wickedness; it was a battle scar brought on by his righteousness.

We need to be careful about how we assign blame for circumstances to the "will of God." We must also avoid answers which subtly communicate, "It's unspiritual to struggle with God over this," because we don't have the full picture. "Life can only be understood looking backwards, but it must be lived forwards," observed the Danish philosopher, Kierkegaard. And as theologian and author, Reg Grant has said, "We must interpret our circumstances in light of what we know about God, rather than interpreting God in light of our circumstances."

Finally, let's explore God's "ultimate will." God created us to glorify Him by enjoying Him forever.[2] We were made to worship Him and have a relationship with Him. Our ultimate purpose is not procreation, but rather to glorify God.

"In the midst of chasing after that seemingly unobtainable baby, nothing else in my life seemed to matter," says Lisa, a veteran fertility patient. "It was a major revelation to me when I realized that having a baby was not the most important thing in life. In light of eternity, life is fleeting. Jesus said to lay up our treasures in heaven. Other goals are not only important, but of eternal value."

Being omniscient, God knew of an infinite number of universes He could have created. He chose the one we live in (with its natural laws) so that He would have the most glorious end possible. This world is the best means to the best end. Somehow this path of suffering which comes with choices is part of the path to glory. We give Him our worship freely rather than by constraint, and He promises rewards for trusting-obedience. Paul, the apostle who suffered stoning, beating, flogging, shipwrecks, betrayal, hard labor, sleepless nights, hunger, criticism, and many other trials penned these words: "For I consider that the sufferings of this present time are not worthy to be compared with the glory that is to be revealed to us" (Rom. 8:17–18).

As we think of life's horrors, it's hard to imagine that earthly sufferings are absent of weight on the scales of comparison with the glory that will follow, but that's what Scripture promises. Paul also wrote, "For momentary light affliction is producing for us an eternal weight of glory far beyond all comparison, while we look not at the things which are seen, but at the things which are not seen" (2 Cor. 4:17–18). C. S. Lewis paraphrased this passage, "All loneliness, angers, hatreds, envies and itchings [this earthly world] contains, if rolled into one single experience and put into the scale against the least moment of the joy that is felt by the least in heaven, would have no weight that could be registered at all."[3]

Is God Really in Control?

Jesus calmed the sea, raised Lazarus from the grave, cast out demons, turned water into wine, and fed five thousand with five loaves and two fish, to name a few of His miracles. In response to those who believe God allows evil because He's powerless to do anything about it, we would point out that they must not be describing the God who revealed Himself in His Son.

Specifically relating to infertility, we find in Genesis 29:31 that "when the Lord saw Leah was hated, he opened her womb." We see from this and numerous other passages that God has power to allow and prevent conception. On more than one occasion we find that God has chosen to open and close wombs in specific and supernatural ways. In 1 Samuel

1:5 we read of Hannah, "The Lord had closed her womb." The same is written of other matriarchs. In the lineage of Jesus, we find infertility in Sarai and Rebekah. God resolved these situations by personal intervention. Likewise, God demonstrated His absolute authority over conception and delivery in the New Testament with the conception of John the Baptist to Elisabeth who was "barren" and "advanced in years."

A Christian patient writes, "I believe God provides humanity with the knowledge to develop fertility treatments so that He might bless infertile couples with children. But I've learned that conception, pregnancy, birth, life, and death belong solely to God and can be controlled by us only to the extent He allows."

Whatever happens to us both in body construction and in circumstances, we know that nothing surprises God. The psalmist wrote: "For you formed my inward parts, You weaved me in my mother's womb . . . My frame was not hidden from you when I was made in secret, and skillfully wrought in the depths of the earth. Your eyes have seen my unformed substance; and in Your book they were all written, the days that were ordained for me, when as yet there was not one of them" (Ps. 139:13–16, authors' paraphrase).

We simply must conclude from the biblical account that God has control over everything including fertility. We've seen that God is all-powerful and that He sometimes causes and often allows infertility. Some conclude, then, that He must be unloving, and ask, "How could a loving God allow this to happen?"

Jesus taught in the Sermon on the Mount that God cares for the birds of the air and the flowers of the field, yet people are "more valuable than they." God not only knows our needs, thoughts, and desires; He cares about them. In fact, He tells us He has withheld nothing in demonstrating His love, going so far as to sacrifice His own Son for us.

Father William Wolkovich, a priest who works with grieving young couples, stresses the distinction between asserting that their circumstances "make no sense" and admitting or accepting that they are "unable to make sense of it." He illustrates this distinction using a jigsaw puzzle: "I ask the listener to imagine opening a fresh carton of one thousand pieces, selecting any one of them at random, and inspecting it carefully. One cannot, of course, make any sense of such a fragment. When the rest of the puzzle has been pieced together, though, one is instantly illumined upon pressing the absent segment into place. The lesson of trust can be drawn from the puzzle example. In attempting to interlock the pieces, one unquestioningly trusts some unknown designer in a toy factory."[4] Thus, some pieces, like some events, seem to make no sense or are downright awful from our earthly, temporal perspective. But somehow they fit perfectly into the whole.

Remember Susie? Today, nine years later, she unquestioningly trusts the "Designer." She says, "God was there. He promises never to leave His children. I don't understand why these things happened to me. I do understand that God allows it and we might never know the reason on earth. I imagine my first questions in heaven will be about why I had to experience two rapes. It was important for me to know that it wasn't punishment or a reprimand. He allows bad to happen, but He makes good from it. It took me a long time to conclude that I'm not going to know why it happened. Ultimately, God's love and power are greater than those men."

God is omniscient; He's all-powerful; and, He's all-loving. He's able to heal infertility. So why does He allow us to go through this? Why won't He heal us? Read on . . . .

For Couples' Discussion

1. What do you think God is like? Is your answer based on experience? Someone else's? On His revealed Word?
2. Do you believe God has reason to punish you? Why or why not? If so, consider praying through Psalm 51 and receiving His forgiveness now.
3. Do you believe God is omnipotent? That He has power over fertility? That He cares?
4. Would you say that the primary focus of your life is on heavenly things or earthly things? Give examples.
5. Up to this point, how have you mentally answered the question, "Why is this happening to me?"

When peace, like a river, attendeth my way,
When sorrows like sea billows roll;
Whatever my lot, Thou has taught me to say,
It is well, it is well with my soul.

—*Horatio Spafford, 1873*

Chapter 9

Why, Lord?

"I heard a story on the news about a woman who abandoned her baby in the bushes beside a jogging trail," an infertility patient writes. "A jogger heard the baby's cries and rescued her. The incident made me furious, and I began to sink deeper into depression. How could God give a precious baby to that abominable woman and not to a loving, Christian couple who had a home, wonderful relatives, and financial security? I felt anger beyond words."

Why do women who hate children conceive? Why don't couples who long for children get them instead? Why do women get endometriosis and premature menopause? Why are some men unable to produce sperm? Why do they get cancer? Why in the world does God allow all this suffering? Why? Why? Why? Don Geiger, a pastor in Indiana, has said, "Often we don't know why, but even if God told us the answers, we wouldn't like them."

Insisting that God tell us why is a form of idolatry. It is, in effect, saying He needs to explain Himself so we can decide if we think He's trustworthy, thus placing the answers above God Himself. We have enough evidence of His goodness to trust without explanations. Nevertheless, He does reveal some of His reasons behind painful circumstances.

To Bring Us to Faith in Christ

Marie ceremoniously threw her diaphragm overboard during her Caribbean cruise honeymoon. She was thirty-three, her husband, twenty-nine. She had all the tangible things most women could want—a devoted groom, her own business, a house with a pool, a sporty convertible, and more jewels than her fingers could show off. She and Mark expected to have some difficulties conceiving because Marie's mother had taken the medication DES when she was pregnant. Years later, DES had been connected with fertility problems and even cancer in the daughters and sons of women who took it during pregnancy. But, Marie writes,

> Even though we expected to have difficulty, we never anticipated the heart wrenching pain we would experience in the years to come.

> We really didn't even try for three years. Then we decided to "get serious" about conceiving. I took my temperature for a few months, and surprise—a positive pregnancy test. We were elated, somewhat cocky. But then I had a miscarriage.

> I was at ten weeks, and it was December 15—two weeks before Christmas. I was a pretty stubborn person, and I generally got my way. I had always bought or negotiated whatever I wanted. Now I slammed against a wall that said, "Some things lie out of your control." That was a shocking revelation. I felt devastated and had nowhere to turn because I didn't have a relationship with the Lord.

> I was not a Christian. I had a rather "eclectic" religious background (a little of everything, and not a whole lot of anything specific). I believed in something, but nothing concrete. My husband and I had promised each other we would find a church we could both attend when we got married, but there were always more "important" things to do. So when I miscarried, I

had no one who could support me with meaningful answers.

My family expressed love and support, but I had so much inner turmoil. Then I got a radical idea: "Honey, we said we would find a church to attend. Now is the time."

I began attending a local church and came to recognize the destructiveness of my selfishness. As Paul writes in Romans, "All have sinned." I knew I needed forgiveness, and I knew I couldn't buy it. I wanted God's power in me to love people instead of controlling them. I found the answer in Christ. I learned that He wasn't just a way; He was *the* way, and His death on the cross provided the only way for me to receive forgiveness for my sins. So I prayed and asked Him to come into my life.

After that, we embarked on three years of treatment, ending with the adoption of our daughter, Michelle. Was the process of infertility any easier because of my newfound faith? Yes and no. Knowing the Lord loved me and praying with other believers was helpful. It still hurt, but there was someone to lean on other than myself. I also began to learn how to give up control and to have more patience. In one sense it wasn't any easier, because knowing the Lord did not take away my infertility. Infertility was not a club I asked to join, but I thank God He used it to help me in many ways.

I thought infertility was my enemy. I thought it was the most devastating emotional trial I had ever been through. After coming through it, I know this—the Lord used infertility to bring me to Himself. Not only that, but also to teach me some humbling lessons I would not have learned otherwise. Now that's love.

Susie's grandparents came to faith through her rape. Marie came to know the Lord because of a miscarriage. Often God uses the closed door of our painful circumstances as an open door to hearing and sharing the good news of eternal life.

Have you placed your faith in Christ? Has your infertility created opportunities for you to share the good news about Christ?

So We Can Comfort Others

I realize this answer isn't "enough." When my neighbor's eight-year-old son died last year, she saw God using his life to draw others to Himself. But she asked, "Couldn't there have been another way? It seems too drastic." Susie asked the same question.

Might there be other reasons why God allows suffering?

Certainly. Another reason God gives for allowing pain is so that, after He has touched us in our agony and reminded us that He's doing something significant in the eternal scheme, we can turn around and offer others a loving shoulder.

"Blessed be the God and Father of our Lord Jesus Christ, the Father of mercies and God of all comfort; who comforts us in all our affliction so that we may be able to comfort those who are in any affliction with the comfort with which we ourselves are comforted by God" (2 Cor. 1:3–4). This verse rests against a backdrop of the eternal reality of future hope.

A woman in our community lost her eighteen-year-old daughter in a car accident. While overcome with grief at the graveside service, she noticed the sun shining on a tombstone nearby. Afterward, she felt compelled to walk over to it. There she found the graves of three children who had died within ten days of each other. Their mother, buried next to them, had lived another forty-one years. She wondered how anyone could survive that long after such losses. Then she thought about the years: 1854–1895. *She lost them for forty-one years, but if they were believers, they were reunited one hundred years ago. I guess I can give God my daughter for a few decades in light of eternity.* This woman has continued to encourage many who have walked through deep valleys.

Keeping an eternal perspective brings hope. It's probably no coincidence that one of the weapons of our spiritual warfare—the one that protects the brain—is the hope of salvation.

Horatio Spafford penned the words you find at the beginning of this chapter. He wrote them immediately after losing his four daughters in an accident at sea. He and his family had scheduled a voyage to Europe; at the last minute, business detained him. So he sent his wife and girls ahead. In mid-ocean, their ship, the French liner *Ville du Havre,* collided with an English sailing ship and floundered. Mrs. Spafford, the only family member to survive, sent a cable to her husband that read, "Saved alone." Spafford started immediately for Europe and, while on the high seas near the scene of the tragedy, wrote this hymn. A century later, the comfort this man of faith found in his God continues to deeply minister to many in times of grief.

Are you seeking the comfort God alone can provide? Are you asking Him to give you an eternal perspective? And are you looking for opportunities to encourage others with the comfort you've found?

To Mold Our Character

Another reason for suffering, perhaps our least favorite, is for our growth in character and faith:

"Consider it all joy, my brethren, when you encounter various trials, knowing that the testing of your faith produces endurance. And let endurance have its perfect result, that you may be perfect and complete, lacking in nothing" (James 1:2–4).

"When a tragedy occurs, we can know that it is only happening because He has a reason behind it," writes Sue, whose baby lived only nine days. "God's loving plan for us is not that we live easy lives, but that we are changed and made like Him. He wants us to be holy, not comfortable. Often the pain of difficult circumstances is His chosen method to grow godliness in us and in the lives of those touched by the tragedy."[1]

Andrea, a patient in Louisiana, tells how she realized she had spent seven years trusting in medical science while seeking God with only half a heart: "Finally, I bowed my head that day two years ago, and I knew I had a choice. The fear began to slowly fade as I placed my hand into the trust-worthy palm of my loving Lord, offering Him my whole heart. Does this story have a happy ending? Not yet, if becoming pregnant and bringing a son or daughter into this world is the definition of a storybook finish. But yes, I have grown spiritually, and I'm learning to trust the Lord. I must continue to hold on tight. But that is something He wanted all along."[2]

One patient has written, "My infertility is not a freakish bad luck event, but a trial God is using to draw me closer to Himself, to help others, and to mold my character. God has a plan for my life. I may not know all the reasons I'm on this painful journey, but I know the One who does. It reassures me to know He loves me and has my best interest at heart. Jesus is familiar with pain and heartache. He suffered more than any of us ever will physically, emotionally, and spiritu-ally; and when He left this earth He sent the Holy Spirit, who is The Comforter." In reflecting on fertility treatment fol-lowed by the death of her infant, another woman writes about how she felt when doctors told her they would take no dramatic measures to save her child's life:

> Faith, which until then had been an intellectual exer-cise, became reality. I felt in my heart that God was not a concept but a living presence. The cold fear left and I felt peace—the peace that comes from knowing, not in my mind but in my heart, that God is present and has a plan. . . . Accepting that God has a plan doesn't always mean we have to like it. The constant grief per-sisted for a long time, and still comes in unexpected spurts. But that morning, I knew I did have a choice, probably the most important choice I ever had to make. I had to decide right then whether to remain

mired in the events of the previous day or to begin anew with my newfound faith and move forward. I chose to move forward.[3]

While God wants to mature us, suffering in itself does not guarantee character growth. Suffering people who have chosen to respond wrongly to their circumstances fill our jails. We have to cooperate with God in the maturing process. We need to recognize our weakness as an opportunity to depend on His sufficient grace, recognizing that He promises, "My power is made perfect in weakness" (2 Cor. 12:7–10, NIV).

Does this mean that once we "cooperate," He'll see that we've grown and give us what we want? In the last chapter, we mentioned how often we hear people ask, "What is God trying to teach me?" It may stem from a genuine desire to grow, but it may also be another way of asking, "Lord, what do I have to do to make you give me what I want?" And it may come from the faulty assumption that "teaching me something" is the only purpose in my suffering.

Should a woman who has endured five miscarriages assume she's "repeated the test" because she's so thick-headed that God had to hit her five times with the same problem before she's learned what it is she's supposed to know? Of course not. Sometimes we limit God by trying to figure out what He's "teaching" us or wondering what part of our character He's trying to transform. We get the wrong idea that if we'll "hurry up and learn patience" He'll put an end to the pain.

God's purposes include instruction, but His reasons in allowing pain are often much broader. In Genesis, we read that Joseph endured ill treatment, not because he needed character growth alone, but because his circumstances would end up saving a nation. Sometimes difficulties may have more to do with how God wants to bless us and others than with our failures. Through difficulties, we may grow to know Him better. At the end of Job's struggle, he says to God, "My ears had heard of you but now my eyes have seen you" (Job 42:5, NIV).

Are you allowing your circumstances to make you softer or harder? Are you moldable, or are you in danger of breaking?

To Eventually Give Us Something Better

In the Book of Ruth, we find a story about a woman from Moab. Ruth and her husband were married at least ten years, but they never had children. They lived in a land where citizens worshiped the false gods, Chemosh and Molech, whom they honored by sacrificing their firstborn children. However, Ruth had no child to sacrifice.

When her husband died, she left her gods and moved to Israel, where she married Boaz. They had a son, whose grandson grew up to be King David. Matthew also records Jesus' genealogy as coming through Ruth. If given the choice between losing a child to human sacrifice and becoming the ancestor of the Messiah, I imagine most people would opt for the ten years of infertility.

Do you believe that if you knew everything God knows, you would choose the same course He has set for your life?

The Final Reason

Still unsatisfied? I was. But after thinking through the "whys," I did actually find a reason that satisfied me. Remember Renee and Marcy, our birthmothers who decided to keep their babies within two months of each other? During that time, a friend asked me, "How do you reconcile this philosophically?" She wanted to know how I answered the "problem of pain" in my own life.

I knew the Lord had used our past difficulties to draw others to Himself. I believed what the Bible says about God using pain to mold our character, and I could see areas in my life where He'd changed me, but all that provided small comfort. I also believed what the Bible says about God using our circumstances to touch others who are hurting. I've certainly seen the reality of this truth, as I've felt so grateful for other Christians in pain who have reached out to me in my losses; but again, that wasn't enough to justify the anguish of our biological and adoption miscarriages.

My own answer to this question came when a friend showed slides of the Milky Way and stated that it would take us a trillion trips traveling at the speed of light for a million years each to explore the entire universe. Then he read these words spoken by God through the prophet Isaiah: "'For my thoughts are not your thoughts, neither are your ways may ways,' declares the LORD. As the heavens are higher than the earth, so are my ways higher than your ways and my thoughts than your thoughts'" (Isa. 55:8–9, NIV).

How high are the heavens above the earth? More than a million trillion light years. That's how far God's ways are above ours. As Paul wrote in Romans 11:33: "Oh, the depth of the riches both of the wisdom and knowledge of God! How unsearchable are His judgments and unfathomable His ways!"

Why have we wasted so much money and so many years and yet still we stand with empty arms? Why did our desperately wanted babies die while millions of women aborted theirs? Why did a seventeen-year-old with abusive tendencies keep a baby who could have had a loving home? *It's a mystery.* In fact, most of suffering and injustice is a mystery.

So in the end, everything boils down to two questions: "Is God good?" and "Will I trust Him?"

In his work with bereaved parents, Father Wolkovich has observed, "To quiet suffering people, I simply stress the mystery of God's ways, beyond our grasp here on earth. Knowing that the bereaved are at various stages in their grief and their emotional and spiritual capacity to accept eternal truths, I suggest that they reflect on the fact that there must be meaning (however hidden for now) in the death of their children, just as there was meaning in their children's lives."

God grows us through our deepening trust of Him in the areas that remain a mystery. As Philip Yancey states in *Disappointment with God,* "We tend to think life should be fair because God is fair, but God is not life."[4] Once we accept that God is good in allowing suffering, we often still err in thinking His methods should be short-term, understandable, and readily applicable in a practical way. They aren't.

Yet despite our ignorance of God's mysteries, we may find comfort in His love and in the knowledge that even this suffering passed through His hands before He allowed it to touch us. In these circumstances, our simple prayer becomes, "Lord, this stinks; I don't understand it but I trust You."

One of my clients composes music for public television. When he heard about our losses, he wrote a song to express his concern and support. His lyrics summarize simply what I have come to believe.

> In the place where no one cries
>
> He will answer all our "whys"
>
> But until that time, we have to trust Him so.

Suggested Reading

Yancey, Philip. *Disappointment with God: Three Questions No One Asks Aloud.* Grand Rapids, Mich.: Zondervan Publishing House, 1988. Compassionate look at who God is and why He allows suffering.

For Couples' Discussion

1. Do you know of anyone who has come to faith in Christ because of your fertility problems? Is there someone with whom you can share about God's grace?

2. Now that you know the pain of infertility, is there someone you can comfort and encourage because of that knowledge?

3. Are you finding God's comfort in your difficulty, or do you tend to avoid Him or go to Him as a last resort?

4. How have you grown through this experience? Have you seen changes in your character and/or the character of your spouse?

5. Life is full of mysteries. List some of the things you find most difficult to accept. Then spend some time talking to God, expressing your frustration and worshiping Him for His omniscience.

Could it be you make your presence known so often by your absence?
Could it be the questions tell us more than answers ever do?
Could it be that You would really rather die than live without us?
Could it be the only answer that means anything is You?

—*Michael Card*

Chapter 10

Infertility:
Does the Bible Really Say That?

$\mathcal{S}$ome people believe that the Bible and medicine belong in separate arenas, holding to the belief that the "sacred" has no bearing on the "secular." They encourage a dichotomy between "faith" and "science," insisting that the two are irreconcilable; but historically, these two have always worked together. In Old Testament times, the priests served as community healers to whom people with rashes, leprosy, or defilements presented themselves. Hospitals actually developed as an outgrowth of monasteries and nunneries. So the separation of the medical from ministry is a more recent phenomenon.

The Bible provides many relevant answers to questions the average infertility patient asks. Unfortunately, some teachers and writers have distorted its message in such a way that it inflicts even more suffering on those enduring the pain of childlessness. In this chapter you will find some of the questions we have encountered in our experience and research, as well as some suggested biblical answers.

*The Bible says, "Children are a gift from the
Lord; the fruit of the womb is His reward"
(Ps. 127:3). Does that mean I don't qualify?*

If God had stopped at giving us salvation, that would
have been plenty. That and anything beyond salvation is
"gravy." God blesses all of His children, but He chooses to
distribute specific gifts differently. These gifts are not limited to children, nor are babies His "ultimate" gift.

*Doesn't the Old Testament indicate that
infertility is a punishment from God?*

In the Old Testament, God certainly used infertility as one
method of getting people's attention. But rarely, if ever, is it
an individual curse. (Michal, David's wife, who laughed at his
worship, may be an exception. See 2 Sam. 6.) In Genesis 20,
we read, "For the Lord had closed fast *all* the wombs of the
household of Abimelech because of Sarah" (Gen. 20:18).

Deuteronomy 28 lists consequences of national evil.
Infertility is one of many items on a list that includes military defeat, pestilence, illness, boils, blindness, hemorrhoids, and mental illness, to name a few. So, if most of the
Israelites found themselves groping in the dark, childless,
sick, homeless, and depressed, they might want to consider
bringing out the sackcloth and ashes.

Further, we need to keep in mind that since the time the
Old Testament was written, God has given a "new covenant"—a covenant of grace. Rather than addressing instructions to Israel as a nation, in the New Testament we see God
speaking and working primarily to and through individuals
filled with His Spirit.

*Does the fact that I don't have a child mean
I'm less spiritual than those who prayed and
got a child?*

No. The Book of Job made clear thousands of years ago
that there is not always a clear cause/effect relationship
between sin and suffering.

The misunderstanding of an association between godliness and fertility has caused a lot of pain, as you can see from

one writer's misunderstanding: "Of the better-known child-less women in the Bible, Sarah, Rachel, Leah, Hannah, and Elizabeth, all finally conceived through finding favor with God. Not only did they conceive, but they did so repeatedly, even at advanced ages, and most of the progeny were sons. In such religious recordings there is a connection with fertility and worthiness. Infertility was a punishment meted out to those who lost favor with a vengeful God."[1]

A closer investigation of Scripture reveals the fallacy of this view. For example, the faith chapter, Hebrews 11, includes a list of God's "Hall of Famers" who trusted Him even when He didn't rescue them out of trials. They endured ridicule, being sawn in two, left to roam and live in caves, to name a few. Surely these people begged God to deliver them, but He didn't. Yet they are held up as the *heroes* of the faith. Clearly their trials weren't brought about due to a lack of faith.

Remember the man born blind we discussed in the previous chapter? The Lord allowed his infirmity for the greater glory of God. Jesus insisted that neither this man nor his parents had sinned. Jesus asked in Luke 13:4, "Those eighteen who died when the tower in Siloam fell on them—do you think they were more guilty than all the others living in Jerusalem? I tell you, no!" And remember Joseph? He wasn't sent to an Egyptian jail because he sinned. Joseph endured hardship because God allowed his trials to bring about a greater good.

In his essay "The Efficacy of Prayer," C. S. Lewis warned against the mentality which teaches that those who get what they pray for are God's "court favorites" or "people who have influence with the throne." Jesus prayed in the Garden of Gethsemane, "If it be your will, let this cup pass from me." Jesus was the righteous Son of God, yet God's answer to His prayer was still "no." In fact, Lewis concludes, "If we were stronger, we might be less tenderly treated. If we were braver, we might be sent, with far less help, to defend far more desperate posts in the great battle."

*Why does every righteous childless woman
in the Bible eventually conceive?*

First of all, not all righteous childless women in the Bible have kids. Anna, the widow who served in the temple at the time of Jesus' dedication, was married seven years before her husband's death (Luke 2:36). If she had children, they remain conspicuously unmentioned. It also appears that Huldah (2 Kings 22:14), Phoebe (Rom. 16:1–2), and Priscilla (Acts 18:26) were childless. Certainly, if they had children, their offspring did not define them or their ministries. More importantly, the Bible is not a textbook about infertility. Its narratives comprise a selective history whose authors have selected stories that illustrate key points they are making.

Let's say an author is showing that the people Israel as a nation experienced infertility when they disobeyed (see 1 Sam. 1–4). Unfortunately, we tend to turn that around to an individual level and apply modern logic that goes something like this: Infertility was sometimes a curse in the Bible; I am infertile; therefore, God is punishing me.

We need to see the author's argument without personalizing what is not intended to be personalized. Dr. John Martin explains the "fertility motif" in the Books of 1 and 2 Samuel: "When people followed the covenant, their obedience resulted in fertility and life. When they did not follow the covenant, they experienced cursing and death. Fertility *was promised to their covenant nation during a certain historical period in their existence* [italics ours].[2]

In these stories about infertile women with happy endings, God was performing the miraculous (granting conception) to complete a special purpose: Isaac, Samuel, Samson, and John the Baptist—each of these and others were born to once infertile women to complete a significant spiritual task.

*Psalm 113:9 reads, "He makes the barren
women to keep house, and to be a joyful
mother of children." Can I claim this as a
promise?*

No. It's not a personal promise. We must understand the literary form of psalms such as this. The purpose of this hymn is not to state promises, but to express praise.

Let's explore some of the context here:

> Who is like the LORD our God,
>
> Who is enthroned on high,
>
> Who humbles Himself to behold
>
> The things that are in heaven and in the earth?
>
> He raises the poor from the dust,
>
> And lifts the needy from the ash heap,
>
> To make them sit with princes,
>
> With the princes of His people.
>
> He makes the barren woman abide in the house
>
> As a joyful mother of children.
>
> Praise the Lord!
>
> Psalm 113:5–9

In verse 7, we see that the Lord raises the poor from the dust. Does this mean all poor people will be raised? In verse 7 we also read, "[He] lifts the needy from the ash heap to make them sit with princes." Does this mean that every needy person in the world will have dinner with a prince? That's what we'd have to conclude if we made this a universal principle, but if we interpret it as a poetic general statement we conclude, "He is the *kind of God* who makes the needy sit with princes."

The point of this section is that we witness God's amazing works in many ways. In certain cases, God raises the poor to sit with princes. Sometimes He gives a barren woman many children. (For example, the two most "fertile" couples in our church are couples who once had fertility problems.)

When interpreting wisdom psalms such as this one, we must keep in mind an interpretive rule. As theological scholar Roy Zuck has written, "The proverbs or maxims are general truths based on broad experience and observation.

These are guidelines which are normally true in general. They are guidelines, not guarantees; precepts, not promises."[3]

Let's look at an example of a general truth in other wisdom literature, the Book of Proverbs. In Proverbs 26:4–5 (NKJV), we are instructed both *to* answer a fool according to his folly and *not* to answer a fool according to his folly: "Do not answer a fool according to his folly,/ Lest you also be like him./ Answer a fool according to his folly,/ Lest he be wise in his own eyes."

Within two verses we find two seemingly opposite ways of handling a fool. Both are generally true, even though they may seem to contradict each other. We use similar generalizations in our own culture every day. Consider some "modern proverbs" or "general wisdom," which relates to how we interact in the kitchen: "Too many cooks spoil the broth," but "Many hands make light work." Which is true? Both are, even though they illustrate opposite truths. We must resist the urge to claim as promises those truths that are wise sayings or stated generalizations.

> *Psalm 37:4 reads, "Delight yourself in the LORD; and he will give you the desires of your heart." Does the fact that I don't have a child mean I'm failing to delight in Him?*

Whenever we interpret biblical literature, we need to look at the genre of the passage involved. Again, in this case, we are dealing with Hebrew poetry, which usually deals in generalities rather than specifics.

Generally, the person who delights in God will receive what his heart desires because those desires fall in line with what God desires. If my delight is in Him, He is the desire of my heart; as I grow in loving Him, He gives me more of Himself. "He will give you the desires of your heart" is not a blanket promise any more than the promises associated with prayer mean I will get a red convertible if I ask for one.

Those who never have biological children have not necessarily failed to delight in the Lord; nor has God failed to keep a promise. At the same time, if God fulfills none of our desires, perhaps we need to examine ourselves to determine whether or not we're truly delighting in Him.

Is it true that the Bible prescribes abstinence during menstruation and seven days thereafter as a fertility enhancer?

Some have said so, and their arguments have included some interesting conclusions: "Abstinence may also enhance fertility. The man's seed would not be given until just before the woman's ovulation. If the man tended to have a low sperm count, he would have the optimum amount of seed available at the woman's most fertile time."

This question is based on laws in Leviticus that pertain more to obedience than to improved fertility. There is no hint in Scripture that a fertility rationale was behind these restrictions.

As medical advice, the assumption that abstinence enhances fertility is inaccurate. In general, the quality of sperm actually deteriorates after four or five days of abstinence because of the dead sperm that accumulate. So, for the couple with impaired fertility, long periods of abstinence are especially detrimental if their problem is related to a male factor.

The same source also says, "The health of the child may also be improved through abstinence. When the man's seed is given to the woman, the strongest seed reaches the woman's seed first. The woman's seed is fertile for only a short period of time; estimates range from six hours to two days. As her seed begins to degenerate, there is a greater likelihood of physical problems in the child."[4]

This author has apparently misunderstood what medical researchers mean when they say that the age of the egg is associated with birth defects. Scientists mean "age" in terms of years, not in terms of hours within a cycle. No conclusive evidence supports the theory that the time from ovulation to conception affects a child's health; but there is great evidence that the older the mother, who is born with all the eggs she will ever have, the greater likelihood of birth defects.

Further, the recommendation to abstain for fourteen days as a fertility enhancer assumes a twenty-eight-day "textbook" cycle. Yet many patients have shorter cycles. A woman may ovulate regularly on cycle day eleven, for example. If so, abstaining until day fourteen would mean she is effectively practicing birth control.

Why is infertility in the Bible always assumed
to be on the part of the female?

It isn't. In the Old Testament law, we find the following laws concerning a practice called levirate marriage. "When brothers live together and one of them dies and has no son, the wife of the deceased shall not be married outside the family to a strange man. Her husband's brother shall go in to her and take her to himself as wife and perform the duty of a husband's brother to her. And it shall be that the first-born whom she bears shall assume the name of his dead brother, that his name may not be blotted out from Israel" (Deut. 25:5–6).

Levirate marriage assumed a male fertility problem. If brothers shared the same estate, and the deceased brother left no heir, the living brother took the deceased brother's wife as his own, so she could bear children. (The word *levirate* comes from the Latin *levir,* "brother-in-law.") We can bet those brothers expressed their opinions when their siblings felt attracted to ugly women; no doubt fiancées insisted on meeting all the brothers before taking any vows.

If the remaining brother failed to "perform his duty," the wife was to go to the next nearest relative, as we see happening in the Book of Ruth with Ruth and Boaz. In Ruth's first marriage of ten years, she had no children. In her second marriage, she conceived.

We would like to think that the levirate custom in Israel never involved bigamy (as was practiced in the Ancient Near East at the time). However, we have no historical records indicating that the living brother had to be single.

In fact, a prominent biblical scholar, Charles Ryrie writes, "Polygamy was allowed in the case of a childless first marriage and of a levirate marriage, but the practice often caused great misery."[5]

This law is based on the assumption of female fertility and possible male infertility. Although childless in her first marriage, it was assumed that a woman would bear children in her second one.

Doesn't God promise to give what I pray for if I believe enough?

Some couples who want a child fear that their infertility is caused by their failure to pray correctly. They read Jesus' words that say we can move mountains if we have faith as small as a mustard seed (Matt. 17:20). They repeat Bible verses such as Matthew 7:7 ("Ask, and it will be given to you") to increase their faith. In each case, we need to look at the context. We also need to keep in mind that Jesus frequently used figures of speech.

Jesus, speaking in hyperbole, told His disciples, "If you have faith as a mustard seed, you shall say to this mountain, 'Move from here to there,' and it shall move; and nothing shall be impossible to you." Have you ever heard of someone literally moving a mountain through prayer? Jesus' point is not that we can make God do what we want by using a sort of "prayer sorcery." Rather, He is encouraging His disciples to pray in faith and watch a mighty God answer.

Sometimes we think that if we just conjure up enough belief, we can force God's hand. One woman recommended that I [Sandi] buy a maternity dress to demonstrate my faith that God would do what I asked. That's a pretty presumptuous suggestion, considering my lack of omniscience and all. The key here is the object (God) of our belief, not the amount. I have no doubt that He is able to give me a child; but without omniscience, I'm unconvinced that it's for my best.

We have to wonder if what we're asking for, even believing God for, is actually what He considers best for us. God in His eternal wisdom is the One who determines whether or not to give us what we ask for. We have to recognize that our perspective is finite.

> *Why don't the promises I claim come true:*
> *"Ask, and it will be given" and "Whatever you*
> *ask in my name will be given."*

The context surrounding the promise, "Ask and it will be given," is asking for God's righteousness. Jesus spoke of this in His Sermon on the Mount (Matt. 7:7), at a time when He was preaching about the internal life and the external life, and the righteousness His hearers must exhibit in their hearts. Later, when He taught His disciples to pray, He threw in a qualifier when addressing the Father: "Your will be done on earth as it is in heaven" (Matt. 6:10).

Jesus' promise about two or more agreeing and "it shall be done for them by my Father" (Matt. 18:15–20) is in the context of the handling of church discipline.

James addressed some reasons why we do not receive answers to our prayers (James 4:3). Our requests must fall within His will, His kingdom, and His righteousness. We must recognize God's omniscience, believing that if we knew all He does, we'd agree that His decisions are in our best interests.

If God continues to say "no" to our prayers, we might feel guilty because the failure must be our fault. Such guilt is false. In his book, *And Hannah Wept,* Rabbi Michael Gold refers to this as the "vending machine" approach to prayer. "With a vending machine, if a customer puts in the correct coins and pushes a button, the desired candy or soda comes out. Similarly, many . . . believe that if they only say the right words to God, the solution will come forth."[6]

"God cannot be bought; God does not bargain with you; you cannot trade volunteer work, lighted candles, promises of good deeds, rosaries, etc., for what you want. This puts God on the same level as Santa Claus," writes a New York City patient.[7]

The apostle Paul prayed for his "thorn in the flesh to be removed" (2 Cor. 12:7–9). Three times he pleaded with God. The Lord's answer was that He had a better plan. He wanted Paul to be weak so He could prove Himself strong through him.

On the other hand, even though there are no guarantees that our prayers will be answered in the timing and in the way we want them answered, we shouldn't let this take away our motivation to pray. Generally, our vision is too narrow, not too great; we often ask too little, not too much.

Is it true that infertility is a curse from God because I listen to rock music?

You think we're joking, don't you? Actually, one source (who also suggests that infertility is a curse from God for using birth control) reads as follows: "There have been several documented cases of couples having children after they removed occult objects and rock music from their homes. The rock beat originated in voodoo worship; its backbeat is counter to the rhythm of the body, thus producing addictive tension. God gives special warning about the danger of bringing idols into the home. . . . Jesus established an association between a cursed thing and barrenness in the incident of the fig tree (Mark 11)."

First of all, regarding the "documented cases," one can find anecdotal evidence to support every possible theory. No doubt there have also been documented cases of couples conceiving children after the wife changed her hair color. As for the backbeat being counter to the rhythm of the body, we would be interested in seeing credible studies which actually validate this hypothesis. Further, in this statement the writer sets up the unfounded premise that rock music is equivalent to idolatry.

This view comes from doing what we commonly describe as "twisting Scripture." Actually, if we were going to twist this passage more accurately, we'd have to conclude that cursing *follows* barrenness. Jesus cursed the fig tree after it was already barren.

But the Mark 11 narrative on Jesus' life has nothing to do with human fertility. In this discourse Jesus gave His disciples an object lesson about looking good on the outside but failing to produce "fruit."

Some of the worst misunderstandings about these issues come about because people have distorted the message of the biblical text. As Peter told believers, "Paul, according to the wisdom given him, wrote to you, as also in all his letters, speaking in them of these things, in which are some things hard to understand, which the untaught and unstable distort, as they do also the rest of the Scriptures, to their own destruction" (2 Pet. 3:16).

> *I have been told that the Bible condemns masturbation. I'm supposed to "leave my deposit" at the doctor's office. Is it really wrong?*

Some have used the story about Onan "spilling his seed on the ground" to condemn both the practices of masturbation and birth control. We read this story in Genesis 38. Apparently a man named Er, husband of Tamar, died. So Onan, his brother, was supposed to take Tamar as his wife, according to the laws of levirate marriage. Onan's father told him to "go in to your brother's wife and perform your duty as a brother-in-law to her, and raise up offspring for your brother." Onan knew the offspring wouldn't be considered his, so when he had relations with his brother's wife, he "wasted his seed on the ground, in order not to give offspring to his brother." What he did was so displeasing to the Lord that He took Onan's life.

This is not an indictment of masturbation or coitus interruptus, per se. Rather, it is a condemnation of Onan's failure to extend covenant love to his brother. His actions revealed the evil intent of his heart. Onan was disobeying a clear command to give his brother a heritage so his name would not be forgotten.

That's not to say masturbation is always right. Masturbation within marriage would be wrong if it were used to deprive a husband or wife of normal sexual relations. In 1 Corinthians 7, Paul specifically taught that couples are not to deprive each other. Masturbation would also be wrong if it included adulterous thoughts, but there seems to be no biblical injunction against a faithful husband "obtaining a sample" via thinking loving thoughts about his wife in an effort to help them conceive a child together.

Why does Paul say "women will be saved through childbearing"?

"Women will be saved through [the] childbearing—if they continue in faith, love and holiness with propriety" (1 Tim. 2:15, NIV). Many experts disagree on the meaning of this verse. Some have said it means that all truly righteous woman will survive childbirth. But there are many textual reasons for disagreeing with this view.

The context of Paul's teaching is Adam and Eve and the Fall. So it could mean that, despite Eve's influence on Adam to sin (she messed up), womankind is saved or blessed (redeemed from wearing the label of "deceived one") through either the birth of Christ ("the" childbearing) or through the role of mothering. In this case, the term *women* would not refer to women as individuals but to women as a class.

Peter stated that sometimes Paul wrote things that are hard to understand. This is, no doubt, one of Paul's more difficult writings. But whatever he meant, we know from his other teachings that eternal, spiritual salvation never depends on the ability to give birth (see Eph. 2:8, 9). We also know that Paul's respect for women is unrelated to their ability to bear children. For example, he continually mentioned Priscilla and Aquila in his epistles, calling them his partners in ministry. When referring to them, he usually mentioned Priscilla first. He also highly esteemed Phoebe (Rom. 16:1–2), without ever mentioning her biological relationships.

Isn't it wrong to covet someone else's children or to feel jealous when someone else gets pregnant?

Do you want *their* child or a child *like* theirs? Does a single man want a wife or my wife? Envy is one of the "seven deadly sins," but don't confuse envy with grief. Often when couples see someone else with a child or hear of another pregnancy, it reminds them of their loss and intensifies their longing. We must make a distinction between a "grief trigger" and "envy." To desire children is good, even the norm. Remember, Proverbs 30 reminds us that it's natural to long for children.

Why do some Christians say IVF is unbiblical,
while other highly-respected Christians
actually perform this procedure?

Many of the differences come from issues of information and perspective. Some of the Christian literature we found was accurate a decade ago, but a lot has changed in the field of infertility in the past ten years. Also, we find deficiencies in the understanding of basic biblical interpretation, as we have demonstrated in the discussion about the Psalms and Proverbs. The important thing is that patients research the issues and study the Scriptures for themselves. (We explore some of these issues in greater depth in chapters 11 through 14.)

Is God good? Will I trust him?

Only you can answer these two questions, and your answers to these questions are the most important part of your infertility experience.

For Couples' Discussion

1. The Bible is relevant and applicable to every area of our lives. Do you have a system of regular Bible study?

2. Choose a time and place and begin spending five minutes a day reading the following: Genesis, Ruth, 1 Samuel 1–2, and the Gospel of John.

Chapter 11

The Moral Maze
of High-Tech Treatment

*I*n the early 1990s in California, the world witnessed the birth of a little girl born through the world's first known five-parent arrangement. A couple contacted the unmarried birth parents of their adopted child and asked them to give their child a biological sibling. The birth parents, who now lived in different states, declined to have a second baby, but they offered to provide embryos by donating sperm and eggs. As the adoptive mother was unable to carry a baby, the adoptive father's adult daughter (from another marriage) served as the surrogate.

Let's assume that current technology had been used in Old Testament times. If Sarah, being advanced in years, was deemed a poor risk to carry a child and Hagar was contracted as a surrogate mother, would the child have been Ishmael or Isaac? Someone actually asked me [Bill] this question during a lecture on medical ethics. It highlights the moral quandary in which rapidly advancing reproductive technology places us.

Then there's the question of harvesting sperm postmortem. The bride of a young man killed in an auto wreck requested that doctors harvest and freeze his sperm because she wanted to carry his child and perpetuate his name.

If we object to the "five-parent" scenario and others like it, do we know why, other than that they "seem bizarre"? By what moral principles do we evaluate such practices? The Christian community must quickly provide some relevant answers, because the fertility industry continues to explode.

America had thirty fertility clinics in 1985; ten years later the number had risen by 1,000 percent. By 1992, about thirty-seven thousand women had taken the high-tech route, resulting in the births of more than fifty-five hundred babies. By 1994, according to *U.S. News and World Report,* Americans were spending $2 billion a year in the quest for a child. The high-tech side of the fertility business has operated virtually without federal regulation since 1979, when the U.S. government banned federally-funded embryo research. Only recently have clinics begun to respond to a law requiring them to keep and report statistics and to be accredited.

Some have contrasted seeking medical treatment for infertility with seeking God and demonstrating faith. As one Christian writer has said, "Hannah sought the Lord; today couples seek a fertility clinic." The apostle Paul himself showed that faith and medicine can work hand-in-hand. He instructed his disciple, Timothy, to "stop drinking only water, and use a little wine because of your stomach and your frequent illnesses" (1 Tim. 5:23, NIV).

An insurance agent asks, "If we as believers accept medical procedures such as chemotherapy for cancer, angioplasty for heart disease, and insulin for diabetes, then can we not also accept that medical procedures can aid infertile couples?"

Fertility Drugs: How Risky?

Depending on the diagnosis, the first move into aggressive treatment usually involves fertility drugs, which doctors may prescribe when tests reveal a hormone imbalance in either the male or the female.

Cost

Often, cost is the first consideration when deciding whether to use fertility drugs. One menstrual cycle on medication can run into thousands of dollars as the drugs are expensive in the U.S. Some couples without insurance go south of the border or to France, where they can legally find fertility medications for a fraction of the cost. Daily doctor's consultations, blood tests, and sonograms add to the expense.

Cancer

In considering fertility drugs, couples must weigh their concerns about the suggestion of an ovarian cancer link. Although largely unsubstantiated, reports of such a link have received widespread media attention and have left patients feeling vulnerable. Further research is currently underway to investigate this connection. Many doctors suspect that the drugs are not the cause of cancer; rather, the conditions which necessitate the drugs cause cancer. Furthermore, if a pregnancy results from using the drugs, it appears to cancel the risk. (Even so, one must keep the numbers in perspective. In a fairly typical study of women on Clomid and Pergonal, only one additional case of ovarian cancer was reported for every sixty-four hundred women.)

Genetic Defects

Some patients have worried that fertility drugs might increase the risk of genetic defects. Concern has stemmed from the fear that pushing follicle development with drugs might increase the risk of immature or malformed eggs. However, to date nothing has shown up in studies, and two key medications, Pergonal and Clomid, have been around for more than a generation.

Multiple Pregnancies

The most likely complication associated with taking fertility drugs is multiple pregnancies, as the medications stimulate the ovaries to produce many eggs. The ideal gestational period is forty weeks, but doctors anticipate early delivery in multiple pregnancies. Carrying triplets to thirty-two weeks, while risky, is considered excellent. More than 50 percent of twins and 90 percent of triplet and quintuplet babies are born prematurely and/or are of low birth weight. They are also at higher risk for neonatal mortality, sudden infant death syndrome and developmental disabilities thought to be connected with prematurity.

For some, these risks are too great; but for many others, what's risky is not necessarily wrong. Is it not worth taking some risks for the priceless pleasure of holding a biological son or daughter?

IVF and Its Sisters, Brothers, and Aunts

If fertility drugs fail to produce the desired results, couples graduate to assisted reproductive technologies (ARTs), such as *in vitro* fertilization (IVF). Approximately two percent of women undergoing infertility treatment eventually move on to use ARTs. IVF (now IVF-ET, which includes embryo transfer) has become more common since the first "test tube baby" born in 1978. The process involves removing eggs from a woman, fertilizing them in a culture dish (not a "test tube") in the laboratory, and later transferring the embryo(s) into the uterus. This is the procedure of choice for patients with badly damaged fallopian tubes, and is often the best treatment in egg donor programs and for couples with severe male factor infertility. The advent of IVF has bypassed the cost and risk of surgeries such as laparoscopies, laparotomies, and tubal repairs.

Now IVF has several variations. "When I looked into the available ARTs, I felt overwhelmed with what seemed like alphabet soup—IVF, GIFT, ICSI. I felt like I needed to buy a vowel," says Melissa, who eventually conceived through ZIFT (zygote intrafallopian transfer). In this procedure, egg and sperm "meet" in glass. Embryos are then transferred to a healthy fallopian tube where they can travel to the uterus.

Couples with male factor problems, unexplained infertility, sperm antibody infertility, and older women are likely candidates for ZIFT.

With GIFT (gamete intrafallopian transfer), specialists mix sperm and eggs in the fallopian tubes. Fertilization cannot be documented, but the advantage of this procedure is that it can occur in its natural environment.

Other ART procedures benefit couples with male factor fertility problems. In micromanipulation, the embryologist attempts to induce fertilization by various methods: injecting several sperm directly into the egg's outer shell (subzonal injection—SZI); making a slit in the shell of the egg (assisted hatching); injecting a single sperm into the substance of a single egg (intracytoplasmic sperm injection—ICSI); and, aspirating immature sperm that have failed to mature and inserting them into the egg (round spermatic nuclear injection—ROSNI). The list continues to grow.

The Obstacles

Specialists generally recommend ARTs only after couples have exhausted all other reasonable options. Couples usually pursue other options first for a multitude of reasons:

Cost

First, there's the financial burden it brings. ARTs can be expensive (ten thousand dollars+ per cycle), and few health plans cover them. Many companies label infertility treatments "elective," lumping them in the same category as tummy tucks and face lifts. Some researchers who oppose high-tech treatment have gone so far as to distort cost figures to further discourage couples. In one study published in a reputable journal, the average cost of a successful pregnancy using IVF was estimated at seventy-two thousand dollars, not including the cost of delivery. But this figure included the cost of all unsuccessful attempts per successful IVF birth, along with the additional costs of travel, lost work, and reduced work productivity, rather than actual dollars spent. If all medical procedures with similar success rates were subjected to the same scrutiny, many "acceptably priced" procedures, such as back surgery, would also be considered too costly.

The cost to those insurers who do cover infertility has turned out to be less than projected. Citizens of Massachusetts have benefited from a comprehensive infertility insurance mandate since 1987. This mandate has translated into four-tenths of one percent of the cost of the family health insurance—many say, a very small price to pay for a child.

Low Success Rates

Others cite the poor odds of success. Clinic success rates can be hard to read. If a reputable program specializes in hard cases, the rates may look less impressive. Nevertheless, experts currently consider a 22 to 28 percent "take home baby" rate excellent. Of 267 programs offering ART in the early nineties, the average delivery rate per egg retrieval was 18.3 percent for IVF and 28.1 percent for GIFT.[1] (Success rate calculations run several years behind, as clinicians must wait nine months after conception to determine actual delivery rates.)

After working through the numerous ethical and spiritual issues involved, Sarah and Mark spent thousands of dollars on an *in vitro* attempt only to discover that Mark's sperm didn't penetrate her eggs. Many couples come this far only to endure the same heartache.

Emotions

There's also an emotional cost. Undergoing an ART procedure exaggerates the intensity of normal emotions associated with infertility. Some have described it as "mental meltdown."

For many couples, IVF offers the last hope of having a biological child; so they face added pressure during high-tech procedures and grief at the end of a failed cycle. For most couples choosing IVF and ZIFT, the main trauma comes in knowing eggs have fertilized and possibly implanted. Getting a negative pregnancy test can be devastating, as the couples wonder where their embryos have gone. Some couples report "bonding" with their embryos and mourning their deaths when they fail to survive. It's important for these couples to allow themselves to grieve these losses, even though there was never a physical child to hold.

Multiple Pregnancies

Again, there's the increased chance of multiple pregnancies. "It felt strange to worry that I'd never have a child while also fearing I'd end up with six in one pregnancy," says one IVF patient.

A 1992 Canadian study indicated that between 1974 and 1990, triplet births rose nearly 300 percent and quadruplets over 400 percent. It is estimated that 60 percent of all triplet births, 90 percent of quadruplets, and 99 percent of quintuplets result from ARTs. Fortunately, with recent improvements in neonatal technologies and services, more and more very small babies survive.

Getting Around the Roadblocks

Couples have limited ways of getting around the emotional and financial costs or improving their odds. There are some ways, however, around multiple pregnancies—but not all of them are legitimate, in biblical terms.

First, there's "selective reduction" (SR). Hundreds of women choose to abort "excess" embryos with SR, an ultrasound-guided out-patient procedure done in the first trimester of pregnancy. Its stated purpose is to increase the chances that the remaining babies will be carried to term, since the risk of extreme prematurity and neonatal death increases with each fetus in a multiple pregnancy.

With improved technology, controlled studies now indicate that triplet pregnancy survival rates are inching closer to twin survival rates. In addition, many multiple implantations spontaneously reduce; for example, one study showed that couples with four sacs had only a 20 percent chance of actually having quadruplets.[2] Nevertheless, some couples use SR to eliminate the inconvenience of having to deal with more than one or two infants at a time. Many modern doctors recommend that couples take risks with embryos and get around the consequences using an abortive procedure. As one biophysicist says, "I believe this is a case where our desire to live in a painless world is clouding our ability to make moral decisions."

Colleene, an IVF patient, conceived triplets. Because she would turn forty before she delivered, her physician suggested selective reduction, but she and her husband considered these children blessings from God. So after spending three months in bed, Colleene gave birth to three "beautiful, perfect boys" who never required intensive care. Colleene says, "We paid thirty-three thousand dollars to have these three boys, and our insurance wouldn't pay a dime; but had I decided to have an abortion, it would have paid for the whole procedure."

Selective reduction brings with it a spiritual and emotional toll. The majority of women who undergo SR find it both sad and distressing to abort some of the fetuses. In one study, a third of the women who chose to abort used terms such as "killing" and "murder" when they talked about what they had done. Most reported feeling guilty. In a few cases, some said it had been even more difficult for their husbands. Some women asked their doctors if they could speak with others who had undergone selective reduction before deciding. Most did not find this helpful, though, as those who were trying to decide had serious ethical concerns, while the women who agreed to share their experiences had found it an easy choice to make.

Selective reduction also endangers the lives of the remaining child or children. Any time you introduce a foreign object (such as a needle) into the uterus, you run an increased risk of miscarrying the entire pregnancy.

So how do we keep from facing such heartbreaking choices? Some alternatives are available, but each one involves some risk.

- First, a couple may limit the number of embryos they allow to be fertilized. To do this the couple may choose not use fertility drugs, so only one egg is retrieved. This can be very costly because it may involve multiple cycles before conception takes place.

- Next, couples can opt to transfer a limited number of embryos to the uterus and freeze (cryopreserve) the rest for donation or later use. But this is riskier for the embryos, and the option of donation raises a whole new set of ethical issues.

- Another option is to use fertility drugs to stimulate the ovaries and to harvest only six to eight (unfertilized) eggs, choosing the best specimens and then exposing no more than four to sperm. Micromanipulation might also be used to control the number of embryos created. In other words, a couple limits the number of potential embryos created to that number the wife is willing to carry to term. Women with uterine problems known to cause early delivery (such as difficulties related to DES exposure) would consider limiting even further the number fertilized.

Regardless of which of these options a couple chooses, they must find a clinic that shows great respect for life. Fortunately, many clinics already restrict the number of embryos they will transfer. For example, the IVFAmerica Program recommends transferring three embryos in women under age thirty-five and four for women over age thirty-five, but fewer embryos will be put back if their quality is good and more if the quality is fair or poor.

The Payoff: Melissa and James's Experience

Melissa tells of her encounter with ZIFT.

I started injecting Lupron in my thighs. Lupron shuts down a woman's cycle so it can be started again artificially. James had to give me the shots, even though they were tiny needles. My hands shook too much. After two weeks of Lupron injections, I started on Metrodin, a potent fertility drug. The Metrodin had to be injected in the hip and, again, James had to do it.

We went through eight or nine days of Metrodin injections. Each of those mornings I had to go to the hospital to get a blood test and sonogram to make sure my ovaries were not hyperstimulated. (If the ovaries enlarge, it creates a potentially dangerous situation.) Finally, our doctor told us we had enough follicles and that they were large enough to retrieve the eggs inside. We had to go home that night; at 3 A.M., I had to have an injection of HCG (human chorionic gonadotropin), a drug that would "mature" the eggs. When James pulled out the needle, I fainted from the stress. This was our last chance to have children. Praying together that night rejuvenated us and gave us strength to face the next two days.

Saturday morning I went to the hospital for egg retrieval. The medical team tried to do an epidural on me, but it wasn't working, so they gave me general anesthesia. I awakened to see James sitting next to my hospital bed. He told me they had retrieved six eggs and would call in the morning to let us know if any had fertilized.

We went home from the hospital that evening and waited for the phone to ring. I couldn't eat because I faced the possibility of another surgery to put back the eggs. So I felt light-headed. Finally, the doctor called to say we had three fertilized eggs.

I went under general anesthetic again, so my doctor could put the fertilized eggs into one of my fallopian tubes. Then we went home to wait for the longest two weeks of our lives.

Two weeks later, I cried for joy when I saw two hearts beating on the sonogram screen.

Why High Tech?—More than Just a Happy Ending

James and Melissa had a happy ending; not everyone does. But even for some who do not take home a child, there is value in undergoing high-tech procedures. Here's Michelle's story:

> My doctor recommended only three to six cycles of Pergonal treatment, and then the only feasible option was IVF. I had been doing some reading on the procedure, but nothing extensive. I knew there was controversy among Christians, but I had never really committed my study to it. Well, it was time for that. My husband and I are both committed Christians.
>
> After doing our research, we saw no reason why IVF would be wrong considering our view of life, the importance of life to God, and our responsibility to obey and honor Him.
>
> Six cycles later, it was time to make the big decision. I had learned that a high percentage of embryos die during the freezing and thawing process. So we knew we didn't want to use cryopreservation. The next decisions came through negotiating with the doctors. We wanted to fertilize only the number of embryos our physicians were willing to transfer to my uterus. We harvested twelve eggs and isolated six for potential fertilization.
>
> We were at peace with our decisions, because we believed we had upheld God's view of the sanctity of life. None of my eggs fertilized.
>
> It was a shock to us and we grieved, but, ultimately, we were glad we had exhausted all our options. We could move on, knowing we had tried everything. No regrets. We were, in some ways, glad that none of the eggs fertilized. It spared us the process of trying and trying again. We felt that God had given us a definite answer to our prayers for a child. Ours would not come biologically.

ARTs: How Risky to Embryos?

While we agree that "a major scientific issue centers on one's concern for human life," we question statements such as this: "Procedures like IVF are wasteful of fetal life and can sometimes result in premature births. . . . Further study and research are necessary before Christians can, in good conscience, counsel others to use these techniques." (We read this in a 1993 brochure titled "Artificial Reproduction," published by a reputable Christian think-tank.)

Let's address some of the errors that led the author to this conclusion. First, there's the premature birth question. The author cites a ten-year-old study indicating that women undergoing IVF were about three times more likely than other mothers to give birth prematurely. Actually, there is nothing about the IVF process which affects the embryos in such a way as to cause premature birth. It's the multiple pregnancy risk in IVF that is associated with premature birth. As stated earlier, by setting limits on the number of embryos being transferred to the uterus, couples can get around this roadblock.

Then there's this statement: "According to the 1987 data from the American Fertility Society, the success rate for *in vitro* fertilization is 8 percent. In other words, 92 out of every 100 embryos do not result in the birth of a baby." Not quite. An 8 percent success rate is not the same as an 8 percent embryo survival rate.

First of all, more current data from the same source (the name of the society has been changed to the American Society for Reproductive Medicine) puts this figure not at 8 percent, but between 16 and 27 percent, depending on the procedure.

More importantly, not every failed IVF cycle means lost embryos. Many couples who begin high-tech cycles find their IVF procedures canceled before the creation of embryos. This is due to a variety of medical reasons, such as the failure of the ovaries to respond to fertility drugs.

Third, the 16 percent figure includes couples over age forty, whose eggs have more chromosomal problems than younger candidates. Thus the failure to thrive may have less to do with the risk of the procedure than the age of the eggs. For women under forty, the average is closer to 20 percent.

Like Michelle and Tim (who discovered during their IVF cycle that Tim's sperm didn't fertilize Michelle's eggs), 20 to 40 percent of couples find themselves facing the heartbreak of no fertilization during a high-tech cycle; but they may be lumped in with IVF failure statistics, even when no eggs have fertilized.

A look at some other statistics helps here. Recent studies in egg maturation demonstrate that nearly a third of all eggs in a fertile woman contain chromosomal abnormalities. Several leading endocrinologists estimate that almost half of all "normal" conceptions fail to result in term pregnancies. They note that most women never even know they have been pregnant because the embryos have died before the onset of the menstrual period. Another doctor goes so far as to write, "I would say that as many as 90 percent of normal conceptions fail to result in a full-term pregnancy. Fully 60 percent of miscarriages are chromosomally abnormal, but it's hard to determine whether as a result of the parents' genetic history or due to a spontaneous abnormality in the embryo."

We do not deny that IVF and ZIFT seem to carry a somewhat increased risk to the embryo, but putting a percentage on that risk is impossible. We know that with "artificial procedures," the uterus may not be properly prepared for implantation. The wife's hormonal support after embryo transfer may be inadequate; with IVF, embryos are transferred into the uterus more quickly (after two days) than they would normally appear in the uterus in a natural cycle (five to seven days after ovulation). This quick transfer takes place because after the first few days in incubation outside the body, embryos do not divide at the normal rate as they do inside the woman's reproductive tract.

Nevertheless, the degree of risk has been grossly exaggerated. Low "success rates" do not necessarily mean we've taken huge risks with embryos. They may indicate that many embryos have inherent problems which prevent them from developing into full-term babies. Not all fertilized eggs divide correctly, and not all transferred embryos will implant. A key difference between natural conception and ART procedures such as IVF and ZIFT is that we know how many eggs actually fertilize in the lab, but when a sperm fertilizes an egg in its natural setting, we might never know about it.

Many who would counsel that "taking any risk with an embryo is wrong," would advise women who have suffered multiple miscarriages to attempt yet more pregnancies by natural means. Is this not taking calculated risks? Some would even go further in risk taking than we would, suggesting that fertile women have as many children as possible, even if pregnancy endangers the lives of mother, child, or both.

Finally, the brochure on Artificial Reproduction reads, "Pastors should encourage their counselees to pursue other less expensive and less ethically questionable options." He cites adoption (which generally runs about two to three times the cost of an IVF cycle), and he fails to suggest GIFT, which at some centers has a 25 to 35 percent success rate. Sperm and eggs are introduced into the tubes, where fertilization can occur. The embryo is never outside of its natural environment.

One procedure that appears to carry a more elevated risk to the embryo is freezing, or cryopreservation. On average, only about 50 percent of embryos survive thawing, though some labs quote percentages as high as 72 percent. Improved freezing techniques are currently being developed.

Some researchers question whether the freezing process actually negatively affects the health of the embryo or whether it merely reveals weakness in the embryo that might have surfaced several weeks into pregnancy. Again, we will probably never know for sure.

Our recommendation for Christian couples faced with decisions about cryopreservation would be to wait until "thaw rates" improve before selecting this procedure. However, we recognize the need for personal convictions here.

The Frozen Chosen: Karen and Chuck's Story

Karen tells of her experience with frozen embryos through several ART procedures:

> When our daughter turned three, we began to feel the urge for another child. While the adoption had been a blessing, I still wanted to experience pregnancy and birth. We had exhausted all our traditional treatment options, so the only avenue left was ART. But both of us had unanswered questions: Was this the Lord's plan for us or only our own desire? Were we going too far to have a pregnancy? Could we find anyone to give us sound medical and biblical guidance? Would any clinics accommodate our belief that life begins at human fertilization? Finally, could we deal with more disappointment?
>
> These were hard questions, but in the next six months, we began to see the answers clearly. Some of the best medical and biblical counsel came from a nationally-respected Christian physician who has an IVF and GIFT program. He gave us specific medical advice about how to maintain our Christian principles while going through very "high-tech" procedures. Then we had to choose a clinic. We prayed, read, and asked a lot of questions. We found the top three or four U.S. clinics that specialized in dealing with our specific medical problems. One was thirty miles from my in-laws. The two doctors there respected our beliefs and felt they could help us. We sensed God's direction.
>
> We scheduled our procedure for November. So in October we began the shots, phone calls, and weight gain. Along with the stress of the technical issues came the fear of failing again.
>
> The first cycle resulted in a biochemical pregnancy, in which conception occurs but the embryo dies within days. I struggled a lot during that time with why

God would allow us to come so close yet be unsuccessful. I had a strong sense of loss over this baby.

Through the procedure, God had given us nine embryos. We had implanted five and frozen the remaining four for future use. When we returned in March to have these four embryos thawed and transferred, I had little hope that any would survive.

As it turned out, the procedure worked. I was pregnant—with twins.

More Decisions . . .

Again, most couples do not have the "happy ending" Karen and Chuck had, but every responsible couple taking the cryopreservation route must make some decisions ahead of time, trying to anticipate every possible outcome.

Sam and Jean, now pregnant with triplets, have five embryos still frozen. Will they donate them to another couple? Will they provide the opportunity for all eight little lives to get a fair chance either via Jean's uterus or someone else's? What if she and Sam divorce? (That has been known to happen.) Will one of them get custody of the remaining embryos? (That's happened too.) What if they are killed in an accident? (Yes, that's also happened.) Have they made provisions for the embryos' futures? Will the clinic decide?

Can you choose to donate them to another couple? Choosing to "donate" one's own embryos raises some spiritual questions. Would any resulting child(ren) be assured of godly parents? Once we have conceived children, doesn't our responsibility extend beyond their physical development to their spiritual development? What if you fail to conceive, but the woman who receives your donation gets pregnant?

Next, couples unable to create their own embryos may want to consider "adopting" frozen embryos donated by a couple who has gone through the IVF process and later decided their family is complete. This eliminates the difficulty of one spouse being more genetically connected to their child, as with donor eggs and sperm. Legally, it's less "risky" than adoption. It provides the wife with an opportunity to experience pregnancy, birth, and nursing. And, more importantly, it saves embryos from disposal. We find it bewildering that some programs prohibit the more "gray" issue of egg and sperm donation, while allowing the more "black and white" of experimenting on and destroying unused embryos.

Couples facing high-tech procedures have a lot of decisions to make at a time when they are under stress and usually pressed for time. We have based our recommendations on currently available data, recognizing that the technology changes daily, but biblical principles are broad enough to apply to whatever technology is developed. Christian couples seeking to live biblically must base every decision about using the ARTs on the presupposition that human life, even at the one-cell stage, has the same moral status as a person. As long as they honor God by placing a high value on life at every stage of development, they may prayerfully choose to use a variety of technological means.

Resources

American Society for Reproductive Medicine (ASRM)
1209 Montgomery Highway
Birmingham, AL 35216-2809
205/978-5000

> The Society for Assisted Reproductive Technology (SART) publishes a report on clinic success rates. Costs are $20 for one region, $35 for two, and $50 for the whole report (three regions). To order, contact the ASRM.

Suggested Reading

Berger, Gary S. M.D., Marc Goldstein, M.D., and Mark Fuerst. *The Couple's Guide to Infertility.* New York, N.Y.: Doubleday, 1995. Detailed medical guide.

Bridwell, Debra. *The Ache for a Child.* Wheaton, Ill.: Victor Books, 1994. Gives brief overviews of some of the high-tech decisions from a Christian perspective.

Cooper, Susan and Ellen Glazer. *Beyond Infertility*. New York, N.Y.: Lexington Books, 1994. Well-researched book. Good resource for medical information.

———— eds. *Without Child: Experiencing and Resolving Infertility*. Lexington, Mass.: Lexington Books, D.C. Health, 1988. Gives couples a variety of personal stories by those who have "been there."

Johnston, Patricia Irwin. *Taking Charge of Infertility*. Indianapolis, Ind.: Perspectives Press, 1994. Helps couples navigate the many decisions involved in treatment.

Questions to Ask about ART Programs

1. How do you feel about creating more embryos than you'll use in one cycle?
2. What is the maximum number of eggs you would want to have fertilized/transferred?
3. What would you do with "excess" embryos?
4. What are your feelings about cryopreservation? What control measures does your clinic have for freezing embryos?
5. Who would get custody of embryos in the event of marital difficulty? Death?
6. What does the clinic do with "extra" embryos? Freeze? Donate? How much say can you have?
7. How would you deal with a multiple pregnancy?
8. What are the staff's credentials? Is the clinic associated with a major academic medical center?
9. Is the clinic a member of SART (The Society for Assisted Reproductive Technology)?
10. How long have they been doing ARTs?
11. How many transfers per month do they perform?
12. What is the rate of live births in proportion to all patients beginning ART cycles?
13. How many patients have had multiple births?
14. Does the clinic specialize in treating your particular problem?
15. Is there a waiting list? If so, how long is it?
16. What is the cost breakdown? What is the fee for cancellation of a partial cycle?
17. Does the clinic have limitations on the ages and types of patients that are accepted?
18. Does the clinic provide counseling?
19. Can you talk with other patients who have been through the program (those with and without "success stories")?

May I adore the mystery I cannot comprehend.
Help me to be not too curious in prying into
those secret things that are known only to thee, O God,
nor too rash in censuring what I do not understand.

—Susanna Wesley

Chapter 12

A Blind Date
with Conception

- Tim and Judy have been trying to conceive for four years—Tim's sperm don't penetrate Judy's eggs. Their support group leader asked if they had considered fertilization with donor sperm.

- Russell and his first wife had two children before his vasectomy. Since Jeannette married him, they have raised his youngest together. Russ's vasectomy reversal proved unsuccessful. He and Jeannette have already worked through many feelings associated with donor insemination by parenting a child who is connected biologically to only one of them. Jeannette wants to give birth; Russ wants her to have a baby.

- Kevin's family has a history of a debilitating hereditary disease. He and his wife, Katie, don't want to risk having a child with this condition, but they long for a baby. Kevin and Katie married in their late thirties, so most agencies will not approve them as adoptive parents due to their age. Their doctor has suggested that they consider donor insemination.

If infertility is in the closet, insemination using donor sperm is buried in the basement. Annually close to thirty thousand women conceive with donor sperm (slightly fewer than those who adopt), yet the rest of the world knows little about donor insemination due to the veil of secrecy surrounding it.

In the not too distant past, artificial insemination by donor was called AID, but because AID looks and sounds so much like AIDS, we now call it D.I.—donor insemination. D.I. follows the same course as artificial insemination with the husband's sperm—sperm is inserted directly into the woman's uterus, but there is one critical difference. The semen comes from a donor. The donor is usually an anonymous hospital staff member or a local volunteer who receives payment for providing a sperm specimen. Many clinics limit contributions to ten per donor.

Married couples use D.I. most often when the husband has an untreatable condition and the wife appears to be fertile. The couple or their physician usually seek to match the donor's physical characteristics with the husband's. These characteristics may include such factors as hair, eye and skin color, blood type, height, body build, race, and ethnic background. In the past, couples let doctors select donors, while donors and couples remained anonymous to each other. Today, more couples participate in the selection process, and some even prechoose known donors. A few, in fact, choose relatives. Advantages are genetic ties, a degree of control over the gene pool, and physical family resemblance. Drawbacks include the creation of awkward relationships, potential confusion of loyalties for the child, and relinquishment of complete control over who will know about the donor.

Anonymous sperm donors usually provide medical and sexual histories. They also submit to testing which should include screening for genetic abnormalities and venereal disease. As of 1994, five U.S. women had reported contracting AIDS through sperm donors. Patients can prevent this scenario by using a clinic that freezes sperm and retests the donor six months later to confirm the absence of the AIDS antibody. Once the donor tests virus-free, the previous six month's sperm is considered safe to use. Frozen sperm do not appear to increase the risk of birth defects.

Due in part to the AIDS epidemic, the American Society for Reproductive Medicine (ASRM) now recommends that only frozen sperm be used rather than fresh, although pregnancy rates are lower. The American Association of Tissue Banks provides guidelines for sperm banks to follow and offers an accreditation process.

Is D.I. Allowable?

Religious and moral issues complicate the decision to choose D.I. Orthodox Judaism and the Roman Catholic Church forbid the practice; however, both Reform Judaism and mainline Protestantism have taken a cautious but neutral stand, holding the position that the decision must be left to individual consciences. In 1990, the Christian Medical and Dental Society approved *in vitro* fertilization only if sperm and egg were provided by husband and wife; they also condemned the use of surrogate mothers. Couples exploring D.I. will encounter a variety of viewpoints. They must answer the following questions within the framework of their own value systems:

- Does using D.I. amount to technical adultery?

- Does D.I. violate the "one flesh" marital relationship?

- Is it immoral to separate reproduction from sexual intercourse?

Is D.I. Equivalent to Adultery?

One key objection to D.I. is that some Christians consider it to be equivalent to adultery. "What about artificial inseminations?" asks Brian Calhoun, M.D., in his book, *When a*

Husband Is Infertile. "Should a Christian use a donor and have his wife artificially inseminated? I believe that artificial inseminations with donor semen are a form of adultery.... Donor insemination amounts to technical adultery, because you take the semen of a man not the wife's husband and use it to conceive.... The use of sperm banks, surrogate mothers ... are surely not acceptable for the mature Christian trying to do God's will."[1]

Another writes, "Perhaps I might concede that D.I. does not involve adultery overtly, but is there a difference between overt and covert adultery in the eyes of God? Christ makes it clear that the sin of adultery is not relegated strictly to a physical experience, but can be experienced mentally and emotionally. Therefore, one can conclude that it is possible for adultery to be experienced technically through D.I."

Is physical contact or lust involved in the relationship between donor and recipient? No. In most cases, the wife never even knows the donor's identity. Therefore, adultery in the normal sense is not involved. We must avoid inventing new terms (such as "technical" and "covert" adultery) linking D.I. to adultery in an effort to then proclaim a biblical prohibition.

Ron, an evangelical pastor who, with his wife, decided to try D.I. says this:

> Some well-meaning Christians rule out the possibility of using donor sperm saying that D.I. constitutes adultery. In the Old Testament, adultery involved sexual intercourse with someone other than one's spouse. Adultery involved a physical act, which did not require sperm. For example, if a couple was caught "in the act" of adultery, they were considered guilty. Guilt was not dependent upon the release of sperm by the male. If a man has sex with a woman but does not release sperm, does that mean they haven't committed adultery?
>
> Next, in the New Testament, Jesus says that if we lust, we have committed adultery in our hearts. The

process of artificial insemination, like a PAP smear, would hardly involve lust.

In our situation, I learned that I had an untreatable condition which prevents me from producing sperm. My wife and I prayed and asked God for healing, which He has apparently chosen not to do. After getting a realistic picture of adoption, we began looking at alternatives. One of our specialists counseled us towards D.I. In working through the moral, ethical, and spiritual issues, we prayed, studied Scriptures, talked to elders, and consulted with other pastors. Finally, we decided it was an option for believers.

"The transfer of another man's sperm to the wife of an infertile man, since it does not involve the third person in the marriage physically, would therefore not seem to me to be adultery," writes Joe McIlhaney, M.D., in his book, *Dear God, Why Can't We Have a Baby?* "Donor inseminations have been part of my infertility practice for many years. I have prayerfully considered the biblical, moral and ethical aspects of this procedure and am comfortable performing it."[2]

Does D.I. Violate the "One Flesh" Marriage Relationship?

Another moral question, which is perhaps more difficult to settle, is whether conceiving a child through D.I. violates the "one flesh" relationship: "The man said, 'This is now bone of my bones,/ And flesh of my flesh; /She shall be called Woman, /Because she was taken out of Man.'/ For this cause a man shall leave his father and his mother, and shall cleave to his wife; and they shall become one flesh" (Gen. 2:23, NASB).

Sometimes there are repercussions when "flesh" from outside the marriage unit is fused into the "one flesh" relationship. Because a D.I. baby comes from the union of the wife's egg with the sperm of an outsider, some see D.I. as violating this "one flesh" relationship. This is different from organ donation in that D.I. produces a new life, whereas an organ is used for the purpose of sustaining existing life.

Those adhering to the "one flesh guideline" generally believe that any technology enabling the husband and wife to produce a child using his and her own chromosomes is acceptable; but any technology which mixes one spouse's "germ cell" with that of someone outside of the marriage is not. Thus, they would condone artificial insemination using the husband's sperm, *in vitro* fertilization using the husband's and wife's sperm and eggs, and even the use of a "host uterus" to carry the spouses' embryo, assuming no other laws of God are violated.

I [Bill] did not have major moral or legal concerns about D.I. when I administered the procedure in the past; but, eventually, I performed inseminations only with the husband's sperm to maintain consistency with the "one flesh" guideline. This was for me a matter of personal belief. I advise couples that this is a matter for devoted prayer and personal liberty. I do not see it necessarily as a "sin" issue, but an issue of individual conviction.

Is It Immoral to Separate "Making Babies" from Sex?

The Vatican, which interprets Scripture for members of the Roman Catholic Church, holds that sex (the unitive) must not be separated from the opportunity to reproduce (the procreative) nor vice versa. In other words, the act of engaging in marital sexual relations without the possibility of reproduction is immoral; likewise, procreation without intercourse is illicit.

As a result, the Vatican prohibits birth control, D.I., and even insemination using the husband's sperm. One way infertile couples have found to "get around" this latter prohibition is to engage in sexual intercourse using special condoms designed so semen can later be removed and used for insemination. In such cases, condoms are considered acceptable because their use is actually intended to aid procreation.

The Roman Catholic Church has drawn conclusions based on a narrow definition of conjugal love, and many Protestants have also adopted their views from this definition. In fact, a writer in one respected Christian publication has said, "Genesis tells us God ordained marriage so husband and wife would come together to procreate."[3] Another says this: "'Making love' and 'making babies' are tied to the same physical act. The pleasure of sex, the communication of love, and the desire for children are unified in the same act. Artificial reproduction frequently separates these functions and thus poses a potential threat to the completeness God intended for marriage."[4]

As we pointed out earlier, God's purposes for marriage and for sex within that union, as revealed in Scripture, are much broader than mere procreation. (See Song of Sol. and 1 Cor. 7.) God designed sex within marriage to include pleasure. As author Ruth Barton observes, "The very existence of the woman's clitoris is evidence that sex was given to us for our enjoyment. Unlike any other body part, the sole purpose of the clitoris is sexual pleasure."[5]

In fact, most studies suggest that only one-third to one-half of all sexually active women are able to achieve orgasm via vaginal penetration alone. Even by altering positions and controlling the tempo of lovemaking, most women need more direct clitoral stimulation than vaginal penetration provides. The distinct differences between men and women in the time from foreplay to orgasm, the refractory period following orgasm, and the possibility of multiple orgasms in the female suggest that our Creator designed us to enjoy sexual pleasure as well as the ability to propagate the species.

While we agree on the importance of obeying Scripture, we question the specific interpretation that leads to the Vatican's viewpoint. If carried to its extreme conclusion, this view would suggest that no sterile man or woman may have sexual intercourse. It would also prohibit postmenopausal women from sexual relations. For this reason, some have suggested that the Vatican redefine conjugal love in such a way that it encompasses all forms of physical expression in marital love, rather than limiting it to sexual intercourse.

In light of this discussion, couples struggling with the D.I. issue must determine for themselves the answers to the following questions:

• Has God given the Vatican authority equal to that of Scripture in determining how the Bible is applied to daily life?

• Is theirs a correct interpretation of the Scriptures relating to marriage, sex, and procreation?

• Can we, with a clear conscience, proceed with a practice that clearly violates the teaching of some churches?

In Choosing D.I., Are We Taking Matters into Our Own Hands, as Sarah Did?

You probably know the story. In Genesis 15, we read that God promised Abraham a biological heir. After finding out "this isn't the month" about 750 times followed by menopause, Sarah got the idea that "it isn't going to happen" the usual way. So, Sarah took matters into her own hands. She brought her maid, Hagar, to Abraham. Hagar got pregnant, delivered a son, Ishmael, and things in the Middle East have never been the same (which demonstrates that the way some people handle their fertility problems can have far-reaching ramifications). Then God appeared to Abraham and asked a rhetorical question: "Is anything too difficult for the Lord?" Within the year, "The Lord took note of Sarah as He had said, and the Lord did for Sarah as He had promised." So Sarah gave birth to Isaac.

Sarah's failure to trust God's promise caused her to introduce a third party into her "one flesh" union. Some have pointed to her error and argued that using D.I. is, in the same way, "taking matters into our own hands." However, Sarah's sin was unlike D.I. in several ways. First, her actions demonstrate her lack of belief in God's *promise* to give her a child (a promise we have not been given). Next, it involved Abraham having sexual intercourse with a woman other than his wife, which is clearly wrong (and which is not involved in D.I.).

Some go on to say Sarah's experience shows that "Christians should never utilize any 'unnatural' procedures, but should 'trust God to provide' a child." We believe we must stay within moral boundaries; we also believe we must always trust God. Yet we would not equate using "unnatural" procedures with "lack of trust." Antibiotics are "unnatural," yet we use them to cure infections. Chemotherapy is "unnatural," yet we use it to cure cancer. One can use "unnatural" treatments and still demonstrate trust in God.

So, can we conclude from looking at these issues that D.I. is right or wrong? The advance of medical technology raises issues of medical ethics. D.I. is a rather simple and, in select cases, very successful solution for male infertility. However, because it can be done does not necessarily mean it *should* be done or that all authorities will agree on its suitability. We do not believe the answer to be a simple yes or no. We must seek scriptural guidelines and then prayerfully, depending on the Holy Spirit's guidance, draw a conclusion that is, for us, gracious and sound.

Couples who feel they can jump over these moral hurdles must then head toward resolving psychological and legal problems created by introducing a third party's genes into the wife's system. The question changes from "Is it allowable?" to "Is it wise?"

Is D.I. a Wise Choice?

Here are some of the primary issues:

The Legal Status of the Child

Not all states' laws address the issue of D.I. children's rights.

An Imbalance in the Marriage

The child would be genetically connected to only one parent. In her work, *Without Moral Limits,* Debra Evans writes, "With third-party or gestational donors, the exclusive marital unity and equal biological bond is divided. One parent will be related biologically to the child; the other parent will not. True, the bypassed parent may have given consent; but consent, even if truly informed and uncoerced can hardly equalize the imbalance. While there is certainly no real question of adultery in such a bypassing situation, nevertheless, the intruding third-party donor, as in adultery, will inevitably be a psychological reality in the couple's life. Even if there is no jealousy or envy, the reproductive inadequacy of one partner has been reified and superseded by an outsider's potency, genetic heritage, and superior reproductive capacity. Fertility and reproduction has been given an overriding priority in the couple's life."[6]

How the Husband Might Feel

The following are social workers' and psychologists' listings of common negative feelings men may have about D.I.:

- Anger about feeling different and lacking mastery over their bodies

- Disappointment and grief over the loss of a biological child

- Fear of seeming inadequate (feeling masculinity is in question or fearing that others will think so)

- Feelings of shame about sexuality, attractiveness, or worthiness

- Depression, which may result in sleep disturbances, changes in appetite, decreased productivity at work or home, general anxiety, and thoughts of suicide

- Considering an affair to confirm virility

- Offering a divorce so the wife can pursue a pregnancy

- Jealousy toward the wife and donor

- Feelings of hatred for the child and doctor

- Mental strain of secrecy

- Estrangement from his wife

One wife, after deciding with her husband to pursue D.I., shared, "He has been treating this issue as 'my thing.' I am choosing the donor. He told me he might be interested in knowing more about the donor later, but now he isn't. I think there is a certain amount of primal jealousy there. I didn't think this issue would bring up subconscious views of manhood, but apparently it has. Right after our first big talk about D.I., he was more aggressive sexually, more removed emotionally, and more into very male-oriented pastimes."

"[My wife] was afraid that I wasn't saying how I really felt when I said it was okay with me to use a donor, and that once she was pregnant, I might change my mind and run off with a 19-year-old club dancer. I did feel a little as if I'd given the woman I loved permission to date someone else. But since the reason was to make her real happy, then ultimately that made me happy, to be thought of as such a great guy," writes, Phil, a D.I. father.[7]

Some couples fear that the father will decline involvement with a child to whom he is not genetically connected. However, in *Without Child,* Michelle Parks writes on the subject, "That was not something that I was particularly concerned about and it has never been a problem. If anything, I think that our infertility and D.I. experience has made both of us more involved and enthusiastic parents. My husband takes great delight in his son; and Jeffrey, who worships his Dad, has already picked up most of his expressions and his mannerisms."[8]

"Our son was born at three in the morning," Phil says. "He looked at me and yowled with a noise like a baby rat, and I knew he didn't have a clue that I wasn't technically his father. From that moment on, the fact that he wasn't genetically mine became mere data. The first time he soaked my shirt and pants with smelly stuff and then smiled right at me, I knew this was my kid. . . . He leans on me when I help him with his homework and his body feels like a part of mine. I know in my head he's not genetically my son. He understands there's another guy out there that helped make him. But it's just data."

How the Wife Might Feel

A woman, on the other hand, commonly experiences one or more of the following:

- Anger and sadness over her inability to bear her mate's child
- Conflicting emotions over what to tell her husband out of concern for protecting his feelings
- Questioning whether her husband is "complete"
- Guilt that she isn't the one with the problem
- Feeling cheated
- Desiring to find another partner
- Social isolation, especially since most people assume women are the source of medical problems
- Yearning to know the donor
- Estrangement from her husband because of yearning to know the donor
- Feeling the mental strain of secrecy

Again, in *Dear God, Why Can't We Have a Baby,* Dr. Joe McIlhaney, writes, "It might interest couples who feel [D.I.] is right for them to know that I have not had any couple express any regret about having undergone [the procedure]. Several couples have returned to have a second child using [D.I.]. Many of these women are long-term patients and I am not aware of any problems that developed for them or their husbands."[9]

The Religious and Social Stigma

How would people at church respond if they knew? Would they say "D.I. is surely not acceptable for the mature Christian trying to do God's will"? What kind of pressure would your child face from neighbors, teachers, and relatives?

Issues of Secrecy and Privacy

What would you tell your family, your friends, and the child? If you decided to tell no one, how long could you keep the secret? If your child developed an illness that required the medical histories of both parents, what would you do? Would your child feel negatively if you did tell her? Leslie, who conceived using donor sperm, writes, "Our child will know from day one that a donor was involved. I used to work in adoptions, and I saw some of the trouble caused by not being honest with kids." Another D.I. mom says, "If we told no one, I feel like I'd be living a lie."

Donor Offspring Accidentally Marrying a Relative

If a man and woman fall in love and decide to marry, what if they discover that they're half-brother and half-sister? It may sound improbable, but it has actually happened. This is especially risky if a doctor uses a local donor to inseminate more than one woman.

Contributing to the "Designer Baby" Mentality

Some complain that D.I. is equivalent to "custom making" superior children. One bank sells only sperm of Nobel Laureates.

The Psychological Impact of D.I. on Children is Still Unknown

Many adoption agencies stress the need for openness, insisting that adoptees have a right to know their birthparents. Yet, it is nearly impossible for D.I. children to trace their biological fathers. Sperm banks are, however, beginning to advocate more openness.

Margaret Brown, a freshman biology major at Saint Edwards University in Austin, wrote in a column for *Newsweek:*

> I'm a person created by donor insemination, someone who will never know half of her identity. . . . I only recently found out my father was not my real father. My parents divorced when I was seven, and I have had

very little contact with him since then. Two years ago, at 16, when I expressed interest in seeing him again, my mother decided to tell me that my "dad" wasn't my father and that my father's half of me came from a test tube. With no records available, half of my heritage is erased. I'll never know whose eyes I have inherited.

In a world where history is a required academic subject and libraries have special sections for genealogy, I don't see how anyone can consciously rob someone of something as basic and essential as heritage. Parents must realize that all the love and attention in the world can't mask that underlying, almost subconscious feeling that something is askew. . . .

So to couples seeking babies in this way, I propose that you find out who your donors are, keep records and let your children know where they came from."[10]

After All That Deliberating It May Not Work

Each couple choosing D.I. risks experiencing an expensive process with disappointing results. Couples may pay hundreds of dollars per cycle which their insurance does not cover. About one in three couples who decide to try D.I. still do not conceive.

Benefits of D.I.

Despite the moral, emotional, and medical considerations surrounding the choice of D.I., many couples consider its benefits to outweigh its problems:

- They avoid a long wait. It requires no adoption lines. Most conceptions occur within approximately six months.

- They will generally spend far less money on D.I. than on adoption.

- They face a decreased risk of birth defects. Statistically, fewer birth defects occur in D.I. babies because sperm banks carefully screen donors.

- They face a reduced likelihood of transmitting genetic disorders.
- They can control the prenatal environment.
- They can participate in pregnancy and birth.
- The wife can breast-feed.
- Children can know about some of their genetic heritage.
- One parent contributes to her child's genetic makeup. Some people consider D.I. "half an adoption."
- Unlike most adoptions, the child may be able to have a full sibling. The couple may order more of the same donor's sperm and keep it frozen until they are ready to attempt another pregnancy.
- They can choose to keep their infertility private. Adoption becomes a public statement about a couple's infertility, whereas a couple choosing a donor can exercise some control over who knows.

"After four-and-a-half years of extensive tests, medications, basal thermometer charts, and synchronized sex, we decided on D.I.," writes a father who wishes to remain anonymous:

> I felt I should give my wife the experience of a miracle that only she can fulfill.
>
> For us, when the moment of birth arrived, the doctor Gave me the opportunity to cut the umbilical cord and welcome my child into her new world. Little did he know what that meant for me.
>
> It will be an experience I will never forget. All I can say is that I will cherish each moment of her life and share her joy and pain, knowing that is what being a father is really all about. She is mine and no one can deny it. The proof will come when she calls me "Daddy."[11]

The Secret Seed?

When a couple chooses to do D.I., should they request that the husband's sperm be mixed with the donor's? This could weave a thread of hope that the child is biologically related to both partners. Yet physicians discourage this practice because it reduces the chances of conception. Many psychologists insist that couples requesting mixed sperm have unresolved issues (i.e., denial) associated with D.I. Others feel couples should be allowed to select this option without facing criticism.

At one time, many felt that a primary benefit of D.I. was secrecy—no one would ever know about the husband's infertility. Marsha and Michael, a rather newly married, Orthodox Jewish couple sought assistance with infertility. Evaluation demonstrated that Michael produced no viable motile sperm. As an only child himself and rather advanced in years, he decided with his wife to elect D.I. when basic studies on her proved negative. She conceived quickly and experienced a normal pregnancy. Their young son was born without problems, and the entire family rejoiced. They decided early in the pregnancy to keep the procedure a complete secret from all parties, and now, years later, that decision has remained firm.

Bart and Anita live with his daughter from his first marriage. Since his marriage to Anita, he has had a vasectomy reversal which has failed to produce the desired results. Anita says,

> My husband has one brother, John, who is a physician in Cincinnati. One day it occurred to me that, if John were willing, he would be the ideal donor. He's married, he's a wonderful person, and he looks a lot like my husband.
>
> I mentioned it to Bart, who had thought of the same thing. Our one condition was that, because we're not on good terms with John's wife, she would not know. In fact, we don't plan to ever tell our child or anyone else.
>
> We checked out the laws in our state, and they say that any child born to a married woman is legally considered to be her husband's child. Beyond that, the legal issues get a little sticky. We talked with an attor-

ney, and his concern was that I could sue John for child support if Bart and I divorced.

We met with our minister. He told us that lots of other couples in our congregation had used donor sperm to conceive. He said one child looks just like her mother, but surprisingly enough, another looks more like her father than her mother.

I've read some books about D.I., and they all seem to advocate telling the child, but we feel strongly that our son or daughter should never know.

Fortunately, it is less popular than it used to be to veil D.I. in half-truths and secrecy. Most literature about D.I. today stresses that family secrets have negative connotations— shame is a by-product of secrecy. Often something that is actively concealed is hidden because of the perception that the truth is bad or undesirable. Also, there is concern that if the child were to accidentally find out, she may never trust her parents again. In addition, couples opting for secrecy risk facing grave consequences if future mandates require sperm banks to open their records.

"For too many years, secrecy in D.I. has been unquestioned dogma," writes a man who was conceived through D.I. but he didn't find out until he was thirty-seven-years-old):

> Today keeping an adoptee uninformed of his history would be considered an unjust abuse of parental power. It is my goal, as an advocate for openness in D.I., to help D.I. parents overcome their fear of disclosure. Parents find loving ways to tell their adoptee the truth without fear of rejection, without fear that the child will not understand. This is despite lack of information about birthparents or fear of a future search for the genetic history. . . .
>
> More and more parents are now coming to realize that their children deserve the same respect shown to adoptees.

In between the old medical position of total secrecy and the newly popular position that D.I. parents should take a stance of total openness, there is room for an "in between" position—privacy. In this case, the parents inform the child of his roots without feeling any obligation to share the truth with anyone else.

Experts disagree about how much to tell D.I. children. Little research is available about how, when, or whether to explain it. However, some therapists recommend telling children at age nine or ten, even though adopted children should find out earlier (D.I. is more complicated than adoption). One psychologist suggests that parents introduce D.I. by saying, "Children come into families in many different ways. Sometimes couples make babies together without any help; sometimes they decide to find a baby that needs parents to take care of him; and sometimes they seek help from a special doctor or another *special person.*"

Children usually reflect their parents' feelings. If parents feel comfortable with the method they choose to create their child, most likely that child will internalize a similar perspective. They may feel some initial anger, resentment, and loss, but if the parents express sadness about their inability to create a biological child together, the family can create a unique bond. However, it is generally felt by those advocating openness that if parents end a discussion with their child by suggesting he not tell anyone the facts of his conception, the positive effects of revealing the truth can be undone.

Considering D.I. is a painful process. It raises intense feelings of loss, confronting couples with their mortality and with their longing for genetic continuity. It is complicated by the fact that male infertility is so upsetting and often evokes feelings of shame and embarrassment. Many couples find themselves D.I. parents without having grieved their losses and without having explored its implications on their relationship as a couple and as a family. Experts advocate involvement in support groups and counseling during and after the decision-making process.

"I believe that if I were to sit down across from Jesus and I were to ask Him if D.I. is okay, He would ask me if I'm loving my wife," concludes Ron, the pastor we heard from earlier. "I think it all comes down to your motives and your attitude. In choosing D.I., was I trying to exemplify sacrificial love to my wife? The answer is an unqualified yes."

Mike Mason, in his award-winning work, *The Mystery of Marriage,* says of Christ, "He was concerned . . . not just to give advice but to withhold it. His way was not always to provide answers, but more often simply to create a climate of moral and theological questioning such that a true searcher could himself hit upon the right answer."[12]

Such is our Wonderful Counselor—He would prefer that we make decisions based on love, which looks different in different circumstances, than to outline everything in red and green with no shades of gray. As He said to Samuel, "The Lord looks at the heart."

For More Information

The ASRM produces an informational list of human semen cryobanks. It is available free to callers at 205/978-5000.

About Sperm Banks and Donor Egg Programs

Available information about the safety of donor gametes is encouraging. All donors should have blood tests for syphilis, hepatitis B, cytomegalovirus, and HTLV-III (which can lead to the AIDS virus). Semen should be tested for gonorrhea, Chlamydia trachomatous, mycoplasma, streptococcal species, Trichomonas, and infection. Jewish donors should be screened for Tay-Sachs, and African American donors should be screened for sickle-cell anemia. In addition, blood type must be determined as women with Rh negative blood cannot use semen from donors with Rh positive blood.

In terms of openness, some sperm banks have identity release programs. When the child turns eighteen, he or she may access identifying information on the donor. Only the child is able to do this—not the parents or the donor.

General Questions to Ask

1. Do you provide psychological and legal counseling?
2. Do you keep a profile on the donor? If so, for how long?
3. Can adult children have access to the donor's records?
4. What kind of information can we know about the donor? Race? Hair/eye color? Education?
5. Do you keep track of the number of pregnancies per donor?
6. Does your sperm bank follow tissue bank guidelines?
7. If we want a second child, may we use the same donor?
8. For what do you screen? Ethnic genetic disorders? Hepatitis B? CM Virus? Sexually transmitted diseases?
9. Do you check the donor's blood type?
10. How often are the above tests repeated?
11. Do you use a donor's sperm before he tests negative for HIV?

Questions to Ask Physicians Using Sperm Banks

1. What is the cost per insemination?
2. How many inseminations do you perform each cycle?
3. What types of legal documents must we sign?
4. Do you offer and/or require counseling?

Grief fills the room up of my absent child.

—*William Shakespeare (1564—1616) in King John*

Chapter 13

More on Third Party Reproduction: Egg Donation

They may be carriers of genetic defects, or perhaps they have no ovaries. Maybe they have a history of unexplained infertility and failed IVF cycles or they're prematurely or postmenopausal. These are the women for whom all other forms of fertility treatment have failed because they cannot produce viable eggs. Now egg (ovum) donation offers them hope.

More than a thousand formerly infertile women have given birth with the help of ovum donation. Most of them have used anonymous donors, and the success rate has run about 26 percent. While many of the issues are the same as with sperm donation, using an egg donor generally appears to take less of a toll on the female psyche than sperm donation does on the male. This may be because the recipient experiences pregnancy and childbirth, thereby making a biological contribution to her child. Also, the process has fewer sexual overtones, as the woman is receiving something her body would produce naturally, rather than sperm. Another key difference in egg donation is the increased risk of multiple pregnancies (about a 30 percent chance) due to the number of eggs retrieved.

The process of donating eggs is much more involved than donating sperm. While giving sperm takes only a few painless moments, the process of ovum donation takes months from the initial screening to the final shots and procedures.

Couples contemplating egg donation usually consider medical and legal questions first: Is the mother healthy enough to carry a pregnancy to term? Does the father have healthy sperm for fertilizing the donated egg? And then there's the child. Most programs require consent forms which the potential parents sign, accepting full legal responsibility for the child. Of course, no one can guarantee the baby's health. Do state laws allow the donor to receive payment? In terms of legal protection, legislation has usually favored the intended parents in egg donation arrangements. No adoption proceedings are required, as the woman giving birth is generally entered as the mother on birth certificates.

The second key consideration is cost, which includes medications for both donor and recipient. The two women must have hormonally synchronized cycles, and the donor must take fertility drugs to mature the maximum number of eggs. Each attempt can cost ten thousand dollars or more (which includes paying anonymous donors up to several thousand dollars), little if any of which is covered by insurance. Can they afford it?

The third consideration is which program to use. Clinics offering the procedure are usually extensions of IVF programs. The questions of travel and length of wait may arise.

Then the couple must find a donor. Medical history is important here. Clinics should screen for the same factors with ovum donors as for sperm donors. However, with ovum donation, there is a slim chance of transmitting HIV. Because unfertilized eggs do not freeze as well as sperm, the same precautions taken in sperm donation may remain unavailable for some time.

Some clinics let couples and donors meet if they want to. In the past, couples sought only a physical match, but today, if given the choice, most will look for even more features the donor has in common with the infertile woman. The preferred age for donors is eighteen to thirty-four.

Some couples ask for or accept offers to donate from relatives or friends. Others want anonymity. A few studies indicate that it's better to use an unknown donor, because it enables the mother to identify more easily with the child and leaves her feeling less indebted to the donor. Other studies indicate that using a known donor has its advantages.

The issue of known versus anonymous donors seems to have some bearing on privacy issues. For example, when a relative has donated, couples may not feel that withholding the information deprives their child of genetic facts. On the other hand, couples might actually feel more comfortable revealing that the genetic mother is a family member, believing the child will feel included in the family tree. Survey research suggests that those who choose an anonymous arrangement may be more inclined to keep the entire process secret. Conversely, those who choose a known donor may be more inclined to disclose the details of the story with the child, family, or friends. Some couples choose another option, that is to tell their child only about the IVF component of his or her conception, without mentioning the part about donor eggs.

While the potential for financial exploitation always exists, most donors are not poor. The best programs screen for motives and exclude women seeking only financial gain. Semen donors have been paid over the years without much hype about remuneration, but the amount paid has been significantly less. This is because the process of ovum donation is more risky, inconvenient, and time-consuming. Female donors must undergo medical evaluation, counseling, and hormone treatments with fertility drugs to stimulate superovulation. Then they endure egg retrieval, which involves the insertion of a needle into the ovary through the vagina using ultrasound for guidance and the extraction of the mature eggs.

Most donors already have children and want to help others. In many cases, they have aborted children or made adoption plans for them, and donation is one way they seek "closure." An important consideration for all donors, regardless of whether it will influence their decision, is the reaction of their families. As with sperm donors, some "donor egg grandparents" have stepped forward to share feelings of sadness and loss about having grandchildren whom they will never know. It is important for potential donors to understand that although they themselves may not feel a particular connection to the genetic material they are passing on, other family members may feel differently.

Before beginning the procedure, the couple and donor must ask themselves some questions: Will the child be "ours" or "yours"? Who else will know about the method of conception? Will it be "private" (only a few others will know) or "secret" (no one else will know)? If we divorce or die, who will get custody of the child? Has the donor considered that this process could interfere with her own future ability to have children?

The Process

The recipient takes estrogen and progesterone so that her uterine lining is at the same stage as the donor's. The physician retrieves the donor's eggs and exposes them to sperm. After fertilization, the embryos are then transferred to the recipient's uterus. If the couple has not insisted that the number of embryos be limited, they may have to freeze some for future use.

The "take-home baby rate" for ovum donation has been steadily improving. In well-established programs, the rates have been up to three times more successful than with conventional IVF. About 40 to 50 percent of donation recipients become pregnant, and such programs are becoming more available.

Some want to throw out the entire process of egg donation because of where such technology can lead. Researchers have delivered baby mice using the ovaries of aborted mouse fetuses, raising the fear that they'll create babies whose genetic mothers have never been born. A black woman has given birth to a Caucasian child using donated eggs, insisting that she and her white husband want to give their child "a better future." Researchers have copied what happens when identical twins separate in the womb— "cloning" or "twinning." Ethicists express concern that a couple could have a child, while freezing its embryonic duplicates. Generations later, the original child's sister and brother could be born.

Again, just because something *can* be done, does not necessarily mean that it *should* be done; and we would agree with those who say that "once a new technology is perfected, it opens up other technologies which are more troublesome than the original. Once started down the slope, it is hard to reverse directions." On the other hand, the fact that a procedure holds potential for abuse does not make the procedure itself wrong. Some people treat sex irresponsibly, but we don't therefore advocate avoiding sex altogether. In Jeremiah 15:19, God encouraged His people to extract what is precious from that which is worthless. We believe that same principle applies here.

Ovum donation involves a wide range of possible uses which may seem interesting to discuss, but our purpose here is not to address the fringe issues of such research. For most couples choosing ovum donation, the concerns are more manageable, if complex. Robin, a Christian fertility patient, shares her experience here.

Egg Donation—First Person

I had been talking to my sister about donating her eggs to me via *in vitro* fertilization, which is a lot to ask of someone. She didn't hesitate to say yes, but I wanted her to know all that was involved before she responded. There would be shots. There would be abstaining from sex as a newlywed, as she was about to be married. Then there would be the hospital stay and recuperation. Add the risk factor. The medications, the anesthesia.

We had previously talked about this with my doctor as "Plan B" in the event that treatment didn't work. He suggested traveling from Dallas to Denver as our final hope. There my sister could donate her eggs to me. The treatments started a month-and-a-half before the procedure. My sister started her shots, and her fiancé went with her to the doctor's appointment to learn how to give them to her. Doctors monitored both of us to time our cycles so they would be synchronized for the transfer. Medications stimulated my sister's ovaries to produce several eggs for the donation; they prepared my womb to receive them. Our timing had to be perfect. We followed our daily prescriptions and phoned each other for updates.

The next month-and-a-half we filled our days with medications, shots, blood tests, appointments, and sonograms. We complained only to each other about our bruises. They dotted her thighs after her series of Lupron shots; I had a hard time getting comfortable at night with my hips purple from the progesterone shots. We both had bruised arms from all the blood tests.

The doctors retrieved seven eggs from my sister. That same day my husband gave his sperm donation. Everything went well, and we felt relieved. Five embryos had fertilized. The other two did not naturally mature and grow. We retrieved the mature eggs; then it was up to God which ones would develop. The transfer went perfectly, and I laid still for the next two days under doctors' orders.

The test came back positive. I called my husband and my sister to share my tears. We decided to send our parents flowers and tell them the wonderful news. In a few weeks, we would find out if we had more than one. That time passed rather quickly.

When we saw our obstetrician for a sonogram, there before my eyes were what looked like three little blinking lights. Three heartbeats ticked away. I saw life inside me. And three . . . triplets!

At four weeks, I started spotting. We went in for another sonogram towards the end of my third month. Our doctor wanted to make sure each triplet had its own little sack. When he came in and said each had its own sack, my husband and I sighed. "Our triplets are all OK," we thought, but the doctor had left the room. I remember wondering why he didn't share our happiness. He returned with another doctor, who looked at the sonogram. Then he told us we had lost the heartbeats in two of the babies.

In reaching for comfort, we decided to focus on the baby we still had. A week later we saw our doctor again. He had expressed concern that when you lose one or two in a multiple pregnancy, the other may soon follow. When we watched the sonogram to confirm the continued heartbeat of the third baby, we held our breaths. When he looked down and shook his head, the nurse silently headed out of the room. We knew. We had lost our last baby. . . .

We had decided to try again, so soon we headed back to Denver. The technicians retrieved four of my sister's eggs, but they called and told us my husband's sample was not good. An infection from the flu had reduced his sperm count. He tried to give again, only to return with the same results.

My sister had just undergone her procedure. The embryologist proceeded to wash as much of the infection as he could to save the sperm sample. The news came. All eggs had fertilized.

Back home, again we waited two weeks, and again I gave blood for my pregnancy test. Then the call came. "Well I wish we had better news," the nurse started out. She'd said enough. I knew it was negative.

It took six long months to clear up my husband's infection. We finally received our go-ahead to return to Denver. The doctor began monitoring my sister; unfortunately, after a month it became clear that her ovaries were failing to respond as hoped. We saw the first signs in her of early menopause. Our doctor told us that if this cycle failed, she would be ineligible to donate again.

He suggested that we try "assisted hatching," which would increase our chances of a successful conception. When a woman shows signs of early menopause, she is showing signs that she is running out of eggs. Often these eggs have a thick coating around them, making it harder for the sperm to penetrate. The embryologist can gently etch through part of this outer coating without hurting the egg, and inject the sperm directly in. We agreed to this procedure. The day of my sister's retrieval, they obtained two eggs. My husband gave his sample, and we started praying fervently that they would fertilize. Again, if none did, we would cancel the rest of the procedure and head home.

News came. We had one embryo. We brushed aside our financial concerns, knowing we had to give this one embryo a chance at life. So the next day we went ahead with the transfer. Again, it went smoothly, but again the test came back negative.

At that point, we had become very familiar with the Denver clinic. We had a conference call with our doctor there, and he encouraged us to try again with an anonymous donor. His wife, the nurse coordinator, had interviewed a woman for the donor program who matched my physical appearance. She called to tell us of the possibility.

During her procedure, the doctor retrieved a good number of eggs. My husband had given his sperm donation; after a day, we learned that we had four embryos to transfer now, and more to freeze for future use. This was encouraging news. It meant that if God blessed us with a pregnancy this time, a biological brother or sister could follow. Soon my days of bed rest passed, and we found ourselves returning to Dallas for the two-week wait.

Robin's experience certainly demonstrates her tenacity, her husband's support, and amazing sacrifices by her sister and donor; and as one of her physicians, I [Bill] shared their sorrow and ultimately their joy.

Not everyone has the confidence, the money, or the time to pursue the same options Robin and her husband chose. God demonstrates His love differently to each of His children so that not all who ask Him for a child receive one. But for some believers, involving a donor brings the answer to their prayers.

Surrogacy

Another option—and a much more controversial one—involving a female donor is surrogacy. There are basically two different types of surrogate arrangements.

"Traditional surrogacy" is used when the adopting mother has neither ovaries nor a uterus. So the surrogate donates both her eggs and the use of her uterus. A physician inseminates her with the sperm of the husband, and the resulting child is biologically related to the surrogate (the "third party") and the husband of the couple. Traditional surrogacy carries with it more complicated issues than sperm or ovum donation because in a surrogate arrangement, the donor has contact with the child through the nine-month gestation and birth.

"Gestational surrogacy" is an arrangement in which a surrogate provides a "host uterus" for a woman who is able to produce her own eggs. In this case, the surrogate receives the couple's embryo conceived through an ART procedure. First, the cycles of wife and surrogate are synchronized with medication. After that, eggs are harvested from the wife and fertilized with her husband's sperm. The embryo(s) is later transferred to the surrogate.

The medical aspects of gestational surrogacy are more complicated than traditional surrogacy, and the success rate is about the same as with any IVF procedure. But with gestational surrogacy, there is less risk of the surrogate forming too strong of a bond with the child or the husband, as the child is not genetically linked to her. Friends and family members are more likely to offer to carry a child for a couple capable of making an embryo together but unable to carry it to term.

In both cases, the surrogate terminates her parental rights to the child, following delivery; and through a legal procedure (adoption or otherwise), the court recognizes the father's wife as the child's legal parent.

The key questions couples initially raise about surrogacy generally focus on the legal risk. The media has provided ample coverage of cases in which surrogates contest their contracts. Actually, of the more than fifty-five hundred surrogacy arrangements, fewer than one percent have involved custody disputes. Surrogate mothers report that they have as many fears of the couple changing their minds and leaving them with a child as the couples have of the surrogate mothers wanting to keep the baby.

According to those who frequently work with surrogacy arrangements, the most important aspect of a successful surrogacy is selection of the surrogate: "The key to successful surrogacy is the proper screening of a potential surrogate to ensure that she is emotionally capable of handling the pregnancy," says the director of one center, who estimates that nine-tenths of all applicants are rejected by mental health practitioners who screen, test, and counsel potential surrogates.

The typical surrogate mother is married, has at least one child, and is between twenty-five and thirty-five years old.

Surrogacy is expensive. Some centers estimate it costs between thirty-five and fifty thousand dollars. Most of that does not go to the surrogate. It covers the fees of counselors, attorneys, and physicians.

Beyond the obstacle of cost comes the long process of matching. After that, it can take several cycles for the potential surrogate to conceive, if she does at all. Another potential problem with such arrangements is the risk of the surrogate becoming pregnant with her own husband's sperm. That happened in an arrangement where the child was born with birth defects and was later discovered to be the biological child of the surrogate and her husband.

For couples thinking about using donor gametes and/or a host uterus, here are some questions to consider:

- Have we prayerfully come to understand that along with the benefits of this procedure come disadvantages? Do we understand what those are?

- Are we rushing into this or have we taken the time we need to fully discuss and work through the emotions associated with this issue? Are we sure we are doing it for the right reasons and not merely to appease our spouse or to avoid guilt about infertility?

- Do we believe secrets are necessarily lethal? If we choose secrecy, are we doing so out of shame? Does a child have an inalienable right to know about his or her genetic origins?

- Have we come to a consensus about how we will handle the confidentiality and privacy issues?

- Can we be open to changing our minds in the future about the level of openness?

- If we opt for secrecy, how will we live comfortably and honestly with that choice on a daily, ongoing basis?

- Do we feel free to discuss this together both now and at any time in the future?

- Is there anyone who can help us work through these issues? Do we need to seek their counsel?

Suggested Reading

All texts are from a secular viewpoint.

Barana, Annette and Pannor, Reuben. *Lethal Secrets.* New York: Warner Books, 1989. Deals with problems that may occur in a family after successful D.I. This book advocates family honesty.

Cooper, Susan, and Ellen Sarasohn Glazer. *Beyond Infertility: The New Paths to Parenthood.* Lexington, Mass.: Lexington Books, 1994.

Chapters on D.I., donor ovum, and surrogacy provide well-done, comprehensive guides to emotional and medical issues.

Cooper, Susan and Ellen Sarasohn Glazer, eds. *Without Child: Experiencing and Resolving Infertility.* Lexington, Mass.: Lexington Books, D.C. Health, 1988. Well-written essays, including a section on D.I.

Noble, Elizabeth. *Having Your Baby by Donor Insemination: A Complete Resource Guide.* Boston: Houghton Mifflin Co., 1987. One of the classic works on D.I. Author's thesis is that D.I. is ethical as long as children have full protection of their right to know their origins.

Organizations

Donor's Offspring
Box 33
Sarcoxie, MO 64862
Donor's Offspring is an organization set up to provide information and support for people conceived through donor. They also try to link donor and offspring.

Organization of Parents Through Surrogacy (OPTS)
708/394-4116
Provides a state-by-state summary of surrogacy laws.

A person's a person no matter how small.

—Dr. Seuss, Horton Hatches the Egg

Chapter 14

When the Cradle Is Empty:
Pregnancy Loss

I [Sandi] ran to the grocery store to pick up steaks. On my way through the floral section, I impulsively grabbed a vase full of roses, anticipating the most memorable dinner of my life. After three years of infertility treatment, I could finally announce to Gary that he would have a new name—Dad. Dr. Bill had told me, "This is the best news I've delivered in a long time, and I deliver a lot of good news."

We revealed our secret to our delighted families. "Finally!" everyone squealed, and we began anticipating how our lives would change.

Then early one morning, I saw blood and felt pain. For the next twenty-four-hours, we trembled with terror and hope as we awaited test results. I stayed in bed begging for God to spare our child's life, praying that my body had not become a tomb, but by the following evening, a miscarriage had crushed our dreams. Repeatedly in the hours that followed, Gary wrapped his arms around my shaking shoulders and rested his cheek against mine as I choked back sobs. I had never known such emotional pain. I felt unjustified in my anguish—I had lost someone I had never known nor touched, yet this loss evoked strong feelings of agony, disbelief, rage, guilt, and depression.

As the years passed, this scene was repeated in our home. The only difference was that, with each loss, our unbounded sense of optimism turned into extreme caution. Slowly we faced the fact that I would probably never carry a child to term as one-by-one each of our children conceived on earth was born only in heaven.

Initially, I found it hard to believe that in the U.S. six hundred thousand women experience miscarriages each year. I couldn't imagine how all these bereaved parents had lived to tell about it, but it was true. Pregnancy loss, though tragic, is not uncommon. While miscarriage can be traumatic for any couple, it is especially heartbreaking for those who have had difficulty conceiving.

In addition to the heartbreak came the confusion of wondering what to do next. Couples who have decided to discontinue treatment often find themselves rethinking their plans. For example, if they conceive on their "third and last" IVF cycle, a pregnancy loss may force them to reassess their decision to stop. The pregnancy becomes the proverbial dangling carrot.

Typically, when a couple faces such a loss they find themselves constantly analyzing what they could have done differently. They chide themselves with "I shouldn't have used that disinfectant" or "I shouldn't have gone camping. Maybe that mosquito bite did it." "If only I hadn't lifted that city phone book." To more fully understand some of the anguish, we need to begin with some medical facts.

What causes miscarriages? There is no evidence that work, exercise, sex, having been on birth control pills, stress, bad thoughts, nausea, or vomiting are responsible for miscarriage. The most common reason for pregnancy loss is random chromosomal problems. Knowing this, people often say, "Miscarriage is God's way of taking those children with serious birth defects."

But at a time like this, logic doesn't help much. It only raises more questions: "So why couldn't God take this child before I found out I was pregnant?"

One mom shares, "In my son's case, had he lived, he would have been strapped into a wheelchair, and he would have had difficulty breathing and digesting. Does knowing this make me feel better? No. Do I still want my baby back? Yes."

Other factors include uterine structural imperfections, environmental causes, infections, blood incompatibility, and immunologic problems. Sadly, one in every fifty couples trying to have children experience multiple miscarriages. As many as 120,000 couples each year suffer at least their third consecutive miscarriage. While a single pregnancy loss is more likely the result of chromosomal abnormality in the fetus, maternal factors are thought to trigger repeated losses. In most cases, the specific reason remains unidentified. Nevertheless, it is extremely difficult to convince a woman who has lost a pregnancy that she could not have somehow prevented this tragedy.

"The only reason not to have intercourse is if you feel you would blame yourself for it later if you had another miscarriage," says one physician who specializes in researching recurrent pregnancy loss.

What are the types of pregnancy loss? Biochemical pregnancy is the discovery that the pregnancy has ceased to develop in the early weeks. A so-called "blighted ovum" occurs when the placental portion of the embryo develops but the fetus doesn't.

In ectopic pregnancy, the embryo implants in a fallopian tube or extrauterine site, necessitating removal, if possible, before the tube ruptures. An ectopic pregnancy can be life-threatening to the mother and is always fatal for the child. Unfortunately, it is currently not possible to take an embryo from the tube and "re-implant" it into the uterus. Ann, after suffering a tubal pregnancy, said, "What a confusing combination of emotions. Everyone is so relieved that I'm out of physical danger, but I don't feel happy. My baby just died."

Loss of pregnancy before the twentieth week is generally called spontaneous abortion or miscarriage; after the twentieth week it's termed a stillbirth. Unfortunately, simply hearing the technical term *abortion* makes some couples feel that their loss is somehow their own fault.

What are the risks of additional losses? A pregnancy loss is generally followed by intense fear that another such loss will occur. Following Nell's miscarriage, she conceived again and spent her next pregnancy "running to the bathroom to check for blood." Katie, who experienced three miscarriages, was so convinced she'd lose the fourth child that it took the birth itself to convince her she was having a baby.

It's not true, as some say, that "lightning never strikes twice." While devastating, one miscarriage does not necessarily increase the likelihood of another loss. There are several determining factors, including the number of previous miscarriages and the history of previous term deliveries.

Although 75 percent of miscarriages occur before the end of the twelfth week, they can occur at any time during the gestation period. Some couples experience added grief because they've believed the misconception that "once you get past the third month, you're home free."

Why do we feel so terrible about it? Depending on personality and background, each person's response is different. The intensity of pain depends on a number of factors, the most significant of which is the psychological investment in the pregnancy. Often, the longer couples have been trying to conceive, the greater their sense of loss.

According to one psychologist, the wave of grief often crests between three and nine months after the loss, although some report that it takes between eighteen months to two years for the scars to heal, and the healing process can be disrupted by repeated attempts to conceive. Couples often feel overwhelmed by how strongly they have bonded with their "preborn" children. Many couples form a relationship with their baby long before conception, with dreams and longings carried from childhood, but a pregnancy puts a date on the arrival. Positive tests provide that spark of hope that allows minds to run free imagining their children at baby dedications, on their first days of school—even walking down the aisle.

As difficult as it is to deal with losing a pregnancy, for some it provides a more tangible loss than having no positive pregnancy tests—the total lack of pregnancy experienced in infertility treatment. Infertility is a drawn-out loss; miscarriage is a compressed loss. In both cases, there is no birth certificate, no lock of hair, and no typical mementos that bereaved parents can stare at and caress.

So once again, we must avoid the temptation to "compare pain." For each person, it's different. Although it may seem hard to imagine, one mother said that by far her hardest of two pregnancy losses was *not* one in which the baby died at four months' gestation; it was the miscarriage that occurred four days after she learned she was pregnant.

People frequently ask, "How far along were you?" assuming that the further along the more difficult the loss. As writer Sherokee Ilse, has observed, "We measure grief by the size of the coffin." Another mom related that the loss of her baby through miscarriage was worse than that of her newborn son.

One question especially haunts those mourning an unseen loss: "How can I stop grieving? If I don't remember him or her, who will?"

The Things People Say and Do

What can anyone say or do when someone they love miscarries? There are no magic words—in fact, silent tears and flowers are powerful sources of comfort.

When people tried to cheer me with "At least you know you can get pregnant—you can always have another," I wanted to cry out, "This is not something replaceable like a broken pitcher; this is a child. I want *this* child." I felt thankful for those who recognized the sufficiency of a simple "I'm sorry."

During our multiple losses, many said and did kind things that soothed our pain, none of which included answers. Those who wept with me provided the greatest relief. With them I felt free to express emotion, so my tears flowed freely. It helped to hear my pal Pam, utter, "This really stinks." Through her tears my mother told me, "We are both mourning for our children."

A Christian colleague said, "Job's friends were great comforters until they opened their mouths, so I'll just say I'm so sorry."

A pastor empathized: "It must have been awful getting that wonderful news and then having it ripped away. I can't even imagine how that must feel. It must be hard knowing you were able to get pregnant, yet not knowing whether everything's corrected for the future."

When an old college friend learned she was pregnant with her third child, she wrote to me: "We are expecting again. I wish I were there to hug you. I know you'll be happy for us, but I know it's painful, too, and that's OK. Please continue to be honest with me. I want us to be able to keep sharing like we always have. We know our friendship is strong enough to handle it."

People brought other forms of comfort too. One mowed the lawn; another sent a long-stemmed rose. Many wrote notes; some called. A coworker sent symphony tickets for a special evening out. One guy baked a chocolate cake rather than send a plant or plaque which might later remind us of our loss. He called and said, "We love you. Can we bring it over and just sit with you for awhile?"

Another couple who had been through the same experience had us over for dinner and let us talk about it.

One note said, "If we could be there with you right now, we'd put our arms around you both and try to share some of the hurt. You know we're here at any hour, for any reason."

And another: "I wanted to be able to hug you and cry with you over this. Today has been sad for me—trying to identify with how you must have felt. Just knowing how I felt was bad enough. Guess sometimes we have to let the tears roll and not try to understand, but instead look at God and say, 'I love you still and I trust you anyway.' I love you."

A Christian coworker came over with his wife and girls for a group hug and Domino's pizza. Tears filled my eyes the following week at work when he asked, "How are your parents?" and "How did your sister take it?" (When I told my sister, a veteran infertility patient, she had screamed, "No! No! No!" and started sobbing.)

"Am I making it harder for you? Would you rather I didn't ask questions?" he asked. "No," I said. "I feel like talking about it, if you don't mind the tears."

"I can handle 'em."

Hugs, touches, and kind eyes ministered Christ's love to us. Others have been less fortunate.

One woman, whose son died three hours after birth, said, "I don't want to hear opinions about whether it was best for me. I need verbal hugs, not advice." When her husband went back to work shortly after the death, several coworkers barely said hello to him. When he summoned the courage to ask why, one explained that he wanted to provide "space," and he didn't know what to say.

"People can't always do what you want," she said.

Some people just can't handle it. They have a certain tolerance for things that are emotional, and when they encounter what seems like the ultimate tragedy, they don't want to open themselves up to it.

We're taught to say "please, thank you, keep your elbows off the table," but we're not taught basic compassion. The things that are OK to say are simple, honest things: "I don't know what to say ... I'm sorry ... How are you doing?" You don't have to say anything else. You can ask one opening question and then listen.

Those who have experienced failed IVF cycles, failed adoptions, and the loss of one or more children in a multiple pregnancy have identified many of these same feelings.

Help Yourself

As with other losses, the way to heal emotionally is through allowing yourself to grieve. Here are some positive steps that can help you in the healing process:

Recognize that your miscarriage is the death of a baby. Life at any stage is precious. Even though your child may have been no larger than the period at the end of this sentence, you were a parent for a short time.

Some may say, "Don't be so sad. It's not like it was a person yet." One mom remembers, "A nurse told me, 'It's just tissue.' It was beyond my comprehension that a thinking, feeling human being would say that."

Here's where holding a high view of life will help validate your grief. This loss is real and significant. Someone died.

With this death you must say good-bye to many hopes and dreams. Feeling as bad as you do is a healthy response.

Find ways to acknowledge your baby's existence. Many couples name their children to help make their identities more tangible. Because one couple never knew the sex of their child, they chose "Chris," which could be either male or female. You may wish to consider planting flowers or a tree as a memorial, or hold a religious service to bring closure. One support organization holds an annual ceremony memorializing children who have died through pregnancy loss. A donation or a gift to a special charity is another possibility.

As with infertility in general, understand that you and your spouse will probably experience everything differently. "I couldn't understand why my husband was less depressed than I was," says Natalie, after her pregnancy loss. Her therapist reminded her that their experiences had been different, cautioning her to go easy on her less-anxious spouse. She alone had felt the life in her body, as well as the death.

One husband explains his apparent lack of emotion: "I believed that to show concern was to court disaster. I developed a private world of superstition that allowed me to believe I had some control over something essentially uncontrollable. During subsequent pregnancies, I was like the baseball fan who doesn't want to call attention to a no-hitter for fear he'll jinx it. I preferred not to mention it at all, for the whole nine months, if possible. I called it 'the pregnancy' or 'it,' rather than 'the baby.' Occasionally, I'd sneak a look at the photos from ultrasounds; sometimes I'd allow myself a few blissful seconds to think about our child. Then I'd rein myself in, not allowing hope to take root. I still leave more unspoken than my wife would wish."

Try to demonstrate kindness and patience, realizing that different doesn't mean better or worse. You each need time to process your emotions. Communication is especially important during this time of stress, so you may find short-term counseling helpful.

On the other hand, remember that both of you are grieving. By focusing on the mother's profound loss, friends often overlook the father's agony. One husband felt so left out that his wife phoned his friends, asking them to drop by his office. Another remembers that people would enter the room and walk right past him to his wife. People sent cards and flowers addressed only to her.

Another grieving husband appreciated the kindness of men in his office who sent a fruit basket with a thoughtful note. His wife says, "It gave him 'permission' to talk about his feelings at work. He works with a group of guys—they're the ones who did this, not the women. That unexpected gift helped him immensely."

As we stood numbly singing in church one week after one of our losses, a friend of Gary's crossed over to where we stood and wrapped him in a bear hug. We both appreciated it.

Expect to feel a loss of privacy. If your infertility has been private in the past, it will be no longer. Those who see your grief will know you feel ready to welcome children into your lives, so your desire for a child is now public.

Many advise couples to keep their pregnancies private because of the risk of miscarriage. One of the most difficult tasks after a miscarriage can be facing people who knew you were pregnant. On the other hand, when you've kept the pregnancy a secret you will find yourself saying, "I was pregnant, but I had a miscarriage." This usually sounds like good news to those who know you've been trying to conceive. You'll find yourself hoping for a little comfort, only to be greeted with an elated, "At least you know you can get pregnant!"

I tried both the public and the private routes; for me, while both were difficult, openness was the better way. You don't have to tell the world, but you should let *someone* else know. You're under stress and need support. Do what works best for you.

Prepare ahead for reminder days—your due date, the anniversary of your loss, and holidays. Expect them to be difficult and pamper yourself a little. Infant dedications may bring even more pain than they have during infertility.

In three years Carol has experienced two miscarriages and a tubal pregnancy. She lost her first pregnancy in March; the other two babies were due in March. She says,

"March is a time when I know I will grieve, and I give myself space to do it."

Mother's Day, Father's Day, Easter, and Christmas, with their emphases on children, can elicit especially painful feelings in mourning moms and dads.

Connect with others who have had similar experiences. You'll be amazed at how many people tell you they've been through miscarriage once they learn of your loss. Go ahead and recount your experience. It usually helps to talk about it with someone who understands. As with infertility treatment, doing research and reading books about what you've just experienced will help take the "edge" off of feeling out of control. You'll find out, once again, that what you feel is normal.

Let people know how you feel. Ask them to listen. Sherril, after consecutive second-trimester losses, recalls, "It helped to retell the details. I wanted to talk about my pregnancy loss nonstop for several months, and I began to worry that everyone thought I was weird. I was glad when friends asked questions. That alleviated my guilt about continually bringing it up."

Another young mother says, "It was hard to find anyone who really wanted to listen. I needed to talk about it but would stop cold as soon as I sensed a hint of distraction or lack of interest. It helped immensely to talk, talk, talk. I needed my friends to just listen and not try to make me feel better. There was nothing a friend could say right after my miscarriage. I just needed to talk until I was done. It helped, too."

"When people asked, 'What can I do to help?' I'd say 'nothing,'" remembers Elizabeth, who gave birth to a still-born baby. "But I loved it when they just appeared with a meal or with rags to clean my house, and I was most grateful for those who took time to listen in the process of meeting our physical needs."

Find creative ways to express your feelings. Do you like to journal? Write poetry? Draw? Play an instrument? Channel your emotions through self-expression.

Recognize why you feel so annoyed when people say, "You can always adopt." You are focused on *this* loss. You want *this* child. No one can ever replace him or her. You're not "there" yet in terms of looking at other options. If anything, a future conception may seem more likely now than before.

Give yourself permission to quit treatment if you want to. You don't have to listen to those who say, "Keep trying. I know someone who had twelve miscarriages and finally had a baby. Miracles happen." When it hurts more to go on than it does to quit, it's time to stop.

Be patient with yourself. Impatience with sorrow only intensifies the pain. Judy wept openly two weeks after her son's death. She told a friend, "Already I feel like people think I'm dragging out my grief and I should be over it."

Years after Beulah's infant daughter died, she wrote to her son, "Emily Jane would have been fifty today." The grandmother of one of my friends took her up into the attic to show her a lock of hair from the child she had lost seventy years earlier.

One psychologist notes, "There's a difference between normal grief and pathological grief. If, after six months, grief still immobilizes them, couples should seek counsel from their clergy or a therapist. But it takes time to heal, and the pain never totally goes away."

If you are called upon to support someone who has just lost a pregnancy, the key here is not to be the "answer person," but to provide time, empathy, patience, compassion, kindness, and the encouragement to talk without trying to find solutions.

A fog still clouds my eyes sometimes when I hum, "Lord, your love just keeps on healing me no matter how I bruise," but I wouldn't trade those bruises. They stand as memorials in my life to my husband's love and to God's faithfulness through the valley of the shadow of death. He continues to bear the burden of our empty arms by equipping His body with what they need to help—tear ducts, gentle eyes, soft shoulders, silent tongues, and listening ears.

Suggested Reading

Rank, Maureen. *Free to Grieve: Coping with the Trauma of Miscarriage.* Minneapolis, Minn.: Bethany House, 1985. Excellent guide offering a Christian perspective on pregnancy loss.

Questions for Couples Experiencing Pregnancy Loss

1. Are we allowing ourselves to acknowledge that this was the loss of a human life?
2. Are we experiencing our grief differently? If so, how?
3. How can we support each other through this time?
4. How long should our break from treatment last? Do we need extra time to "work through" our pain?
5. Would it help for us to tangibly acknowledge our baby's existence through holding a memorial service? By planting a tree? Some other way?

Resources for Couples Experiencing Pregnancy Loss

The Compassionate Friends
P.O. Box 3696
Oak Brook, IL 60522-3696
708/990-0010
> Self-help group for bereaved parents who have lost children of any age. Local chapters.

Our Newsletter
P.O. Box 1064
Palmer, Alaska 99645
> Offers newsletter for those grieving the loss of one or more children in a multiple birth.

Pen Parents
P.O. Box 8738
Reno, NV 89507-8738
702/826-7332
> Provides newsletter for families who have experienced neonatal loss.

RESOLVE
1310 Broadway
Somerville, MA 92144-1731
617/623-0744
> Provides fact sheets, referral, support, and advocacy.

SHARE: Pregnancy and Infant Loss Support, Inc.
c/o St. Joseph's Health Center
300 First Capital Drive
St. Charles, MO 63301
314/947-5000
> Through local chapters, helps parents deal with miscarriage, stillbirth, or neonatal loss.

Nobody knows the trouble I've seen.
Nobody knows but Jesus.

Chapter 15

Execution or Empathy?
For Those Who Parent

$\mathcal{M}$ention secondary infertility and many people (including many "primary" couples) say, "At least they have one. . . ."

A woman who is pregnant after infertility asks if she can still attend her infertility support group because she has so many fears. She hears, "No way. We don't want to see that fat belly. . . ."

A new adoptive father verbalizes his need for more sleep. His words are met with, "If I had a child, I would be thankful for those cries that kept me up."

When we read the Gospel of Luke, we see two cousins who are facing very different situations, both of them relating to having children. Elisabeth, wife of Zacharias, has spent years feeling ashamed of her infertility. Mary, the unmarried mother of Jesus, learns that she will soon bear a child. Both women face some adjustments. Do you suppose anyone said to Mary, "Well, you may have to face some public shame, but at least you don't have to deal with the embarrassment Elisabeth has had to handle all these years"? I hope not.

Comparing "stuff" almost always gets us into trouble. So often as we infertile couples stand crying for someone to acknowledge our pain, we walk coldly away from others we deem more fortunate. The very things we beg for—empathy, compassion, understanding, and grace—we refuse to give. So let's take a look at some situations in which we may need to sharpen our "empathy radar."

Secondary Infertility

When Margo and Larry tried to have a second child, they were shocked to discover they had a fertility problem. "Our profound disappointment has taken its toll on our marriage and even on our child," says Margo. "When I look at the empty chair at the dinner table, I feel like someone is missing."

Margo and Larry have plenty of company. Couples with one or more children experience infertility even more commonly than couples with no children. These may be couples for whom pregnancy came easily the first time, or infertility may have plagued their first attempt at pregnancy and is resurfacing as they try again to conceive. (In the latter case, the couple is actually having primary infertility the second time around.)

Secondary infertility seems to be undertreated. Research reveals that while half of all couples diagnosed with primary infertility pursue treatment, only one-fifth of couples with secondary infertility seek medical help. Of those who do, close to half will eventually bear another child. For those who don't pursue treatment, the percentage drops to five.

Primary and secondary infertility patients experience almost identical medical problems and treatments. In addition, childbirth can cause some fertility problems, such as infection and scarring; naturally, couples are older when they try to have children again. The chances of conceiving per cycle drop off drastically in the upper thirties. So couples can't assume everything is all right because they've previously had a child.

Primary and secondary infertility are also similar emotionally. Psychologists confirm that both evoke feelings of guilt, denial, anger, depression, and frustration. But differences exist, too. Secondary infertile couples are at an in-between place. The *fertile* population perceives them as having no fertility problem because they've conceived. Yet when they are among the *infertile* population, they feel too ashamed to ask for support for fear childless couples will resent them.

Debra, who is seeking treatment after having a "miracle baby," says the second time she feels a different kind of pain. "Now that I have one child, there's a new ache. I've exchanged the anguish of having no child for the pain of knowing exactly what I'm missing the second time, and a child can cause barriers. I feel like the people to whom I used to run for comfort no longer accept me as 'one of them.'"

Many parents worry that their deep desire to have a second child will scar their existing child. They feel sad and go to the doctor a lot. Does their child worry that Mom and Dad are dying? They avoid situations where infants are present. Will their child conclude that babies are bad? They argued about babies last night. Does their son think he is not good enough? Does their daughter think they don't love each other anymore?

Another young mom finds that having a child throws her into a world where it's harder to protect herself. An activity as common as picking up her daughter from nursery school brings unexpected grief: "You notice you're the only mother who is not visibly pregnant, carrying an infant, or holding a toddler's hand," she says. She goes on to add, "Your kindergartner asks why she's the only child in her class with no brothers or sisters. You listen to everyone in your play group discuss how far apart they want to space their children, and then, incredibly, you watch them give birth exactly according to plan. Meanwhile, you continue with temperature charts, medications, and endless doctor visits. You struggle politely to answer unsuspecting friends and relatives who comment, 'Time for another, isn't it?' Or worse, those in whom you've confided that you're infertile tell you, 'At least you have one child; you should feel grateful.'"

"It's nearly impossible to explain to someone who feels their family is complete why you desire so strongly and actually grieve for the 'phantom child,'" says Margo. "Well-meaning people try to tell us we should feel satisfied with the child we have. I compare it to how I feel about my mother. She died a few months before my baby was born. Eventually I was able to feel grateful to God for giving me a wonderful mother and to Mom for being such a good mother. But no matter how grateful I felt, it never took away my longing to be with her, talk to her, and hug her. Gratitude will never replace that longing, just as gratitude for the child I have will never replace my longing for another child."

Patti finds herself back in treatment after giving birth two years ago. She talks frequently with other women experiencing secondary infertility, and observes, "A loss is a loss. Childbirth doesn't take away the desire to be a mother again. Once you've felt something—something wonderful—and it's taken away, it leaves an aching emptiness inside."

Another compares the feeling of being "grateful" to an amputee. "If you have one leg, of course, you're grateful, but having two would certainly be better."

Secondary infertility brings with it an overwhelming jolt—the realization that dreams may never materialize. One mother says, "Many of us grew up with a vision that our ideal family would consist of at least two children. I think about my daughter and wonder if she will ever know the mischief of sisters caught with Mom's makeup, the frustration of having to share her toys, and the confidences that can't bridge generations. When we get old and start acting funny, who will she call to say, 'How can we keep Dad from climbing ladders to clean gutters?' or 'We've got to get Mom to stop wearing T-shirts to Neiman-Marcus.' I watch her now with two sets of eyes. One set watches her as any mother would. The other struggles to memorize every stage."

Another mother explains her compelling need to savor each moment: "I know I have many happy years ahead with my daughter, but I'm having a hard time accepting that I will experience these things only once."

Daniel's mother, like most, feels guilty about her inability to give her son a sister or a brother, recounting a recent experience that made her cry: "The neighbor kids were teasing my son, saying 'If we didn't live next door, you'd have nobody to play with. Ha! Ha! You don't have any brothers or sisters.' I called their mother, and she told me her kids felt jealous because my son had more toys. She and her husband told their children to consider themselves lucky. While Daniel had lots of toys, they had brothers and sisters something Daniel didn't have."

Another mom, when describing how her son brought home a book and asked her to read it to him remembers, "I almost lost it." The title: *Spot's Baby Sister.*

"My daughter, who was adopted, has told everyone in her day-care center that I'm expecting," says Susan, whose little girl is four. "It's so awkward to explain to everyone that I'm not! But the topper was when she told me, 'I have a tummy ache. I think I'm pregnant.'" Then come the fears. Many parents fear that their "only children" will be lonely, lacking family connections. They may become overly protective or unusually ambitious for their single child. They also worry that their child will die or bear the sole burden of caring for them in their old age. Studies show that only children tend to be self-starters who are confident and rank high in intelligence, and they experience less jealousy and engage in less sexual stereotyping than do children with siblings. But while there are benefits, the pressure to be a successful parent is increased with an only child.

Guilt may enter the picture. Studies show that many moms and dads with fertility problems harangue themselves about the quality of their parenting. They may wonder if God is punishing them for being imperfect parents the first time. When their child misbehaves, they may think, "We can't even raise this one right. No wonder we're not supposed to have another!"

They may also have feelings of regret, especially the mother, who may now wish she had savored the experience of childbirth more, cherishing every moment of pregnancy. Often couples find themselves explaining that they *want* more children. They hear hints that they are being "selfish" to deprive their child of a sibling or they field inquiries about why they've sacrificed a larger family for high-powered careers.

Mary shares, "After I had several miscarriages, my husband had a vasectomy; but we just moved to a community where many of the people don't believe in birth control. When they see our family of four (one adopted, one biological child), they wonder when I'll have more children. They tend to assess spirituality in terms of home schooling, organic gardening, and the number of children we have rather than by the fruit of the Spirit. Talk about pressure."

Frequently couples face marital strain, especially when one partner, usually the female, feels more strongly about having additional children. After the birth of the first child, many men find that their parenting needs are fulfilled, say Helane S. Rosenberg, Ph.D., and Yakov M. Epstein, Ph.D, authors of *Getting Pregnant When You Thought You Couldn't.* Women, on the other hand, may have an entirely different image of family size. For a lot of men, a second child is desirable, but not critical. So a woman yearning for more children may lose her husband's support at a time when she has also lost the encouragement of friends, relatives, physicians, and primary infertility patients.

Many couples find that secondary infertility can also complicate the adoption question. They worry about real or perceived equality in homes with a biological/adoptive mix. Some agencies turn away couples with a biological child, and many have a ceiling on parental age. Couples confronting secondary infertility need empathy and validation of their pain. They need the freedom to grieve their many losses, and they need support in resolving their crises.

Stacia, describing the emptiness she feels over being unable to conceive again, says, "This is the most difficult thing I've ever dealt with. A nurse once told me, 'Secondary infertility is like getting up from the dinner table when you're still hungry.' She was right. I know I will always feel like I'm just not finished."

Pregnancy after Infertility

"I always thought that pregnancy after infertility must be incredible, joyous, and thrilling. It was the dream I had long since given up on. Then I received a positive pregnancy test. I quickly discovered that the words *pregnancy after infertility* were more complex than I ever could have imagined," writes Elana. "I was not feeling joyous or thrilled, but skeptical, angry, and scared. While I had come to know and accept my role as an infertile woman, I now felt like an impostor as a pregnant one."

As we infertility patients make our daily runs to the lab, we tend to focus on a positive pregnancy test as the ultimate end to our infertility, visualizing the inauguration of a nine-month celebration. So when the great news actually comes, we find ourselves unprepared for the stress.

Most infertility patients have become programmed for failure. So it's hard to believe, even after a positive test, that "all is well." Elana continues, "I anticipated bad news even after the positive test, since bad news had become so familiar to me."

Next, they may find themselves defined as "regular" patients in busy obstetrical practices. Coming from situations in which they may know the entire medical staff by name, patients have often received a lot of special attention. But now they are told, "Come back again in six weeks." The new practice seems to lack any sense of urgency.

Also, pregnant patients often feel unwelcome in the world of the infertile, but they identify more with that world. The fertile world seems too carefree, too unappreciative of what is at stake here. "I am not a member of the 'fertile club,'" writes an expectant father. "My wife and I cannot 'just have another.' This was our one last shot, but I am no longer a true member of the 'infertile club,' either. I am, in a word, nowhere."

If you find yourself experiencing pregnancy after infertility, you probably will not feel that normal freedom to heartily agree with complaints such as "I hate it when the baby makes my bladder feel like it's the size of a lentil." Instead, you will probably expect yourself to have an attitude more like, "Every barf a blessing." Yet other pregnant women will see that you have something in common and will confide in you about their aches, pains, and fears about the risks of C-section deliveries. "I feel like a fake," one expectant mother confessed. "I'm having trouble integrating pregnancy into my identity."

Some patients find that their feelings about looking pregnant change. Before they conceived, they may have secretly promised themselves that they'd be thrilled over every body change related to carrying a child; but those who have spent two or three decades taking pride in trim figures report a harder-than-expected adjustment to their new size.

Then there's the fear of pregnancy loss and birth defects. "We lost one of the babies in a triplet pregnancy," says one mother. "I stayed on edge awaiting disaster after that."

One expectant father likens his experience to "survivor guilt":

> In no small measure, my guilt is mixed with loneliness. I have moved forward, where others are left behind. I have prospered, where others are impoverished. In a very real sense, I cannot understand why I should be the lucky one. I had thought that once my family was on the way, I would feel only happiness. And I do. But I feel cheated out of that total joy that fertile couples feel. It is funny that I feel this guilt for something that alternately sends me soaring and crashing, but I want my friends to soar with me so we can share

in that elation. And I want my friends to be with me during those dark times of fear and doubt. Just as my infertility is, so is my happiness unfair.[1]

Parenting after Infertility

Leigh writes this four months after the arrival of her miracle baby:

> I feel awful that I can't give this happiness to every infertile person. Yet I feel unwelcome and unwanted. Mine is a sad, lonely place. I walk down the street wondering who wants to throw a rock at me because I have a child. Do they even know I spent years trying to conceive him? That I lost his sibling to miscarriage before him? No. And do they care? I still feel hurt when someone announces her pregnancy, even though I have my miracle. Having a baby does not make you forget and, in my case, does not take that longing and sad infertility feeling away. Yes, I am hurting too.

Inevitably, the question comes up about having a second child. Often people ask, "When do you plan to have another?" If you've spent fifty thousand dollars the first time around, you may have no resources left. Advancing age can leave few options here. Planning for a second child has made some mothers stop nursing so it won't interfere with treatment. "I feel like I don't have time to enjoy the child I finally have because we have so little time," says one despairing mother who thought her anxiety would end with pregnancy. She worries that she will be overprotective with her one "miracle baby."

Many infertile parents find themselves feeling a little disappointment when "it's all over" and they have their "happy ending." The adjustment to parenthood brings stress to the most stable of marital relationships. Sleep deprivation, especially for parents of multiples, can make you wonder if you made a mistake.

Remember "Julia Child . . . less"? She wrote this to explain her feelings about finally being a parent:

I thought that when I finally became a parent at long last I could resume life as a normal person. Infertility was behind me, normal parenthood ahead, but infertility's legacy has blocked my ability to be a normal parent. Instead of being somewhat comfortable with the usual ambivalent emotions that average mothers feel toward their children, I feel guilty.

Ellen Glazer, an infertility author, refers to it as "being eternally grateful." When I find myself angry at my child, I feel awful. When on a bad day I think to myself, Today I wish I didn't have a child, I expect a lightning bolt to strike in my living room. So far, no lightning bolts, but lots of guilt.

Ambivalent feelings are what parenthood is all about. She smiles at you, and it melts your heart. Then she spits peas on your white silk blouse and you want to kill her. I think fertile parents take these ambivalent feelings in stride, but not so if you're infertile. Wanting to "kill" your child does not fit well with being "eternally grateful."

"If you wanted this child so much, how could you possibly hate her at this moment?" "If you really love her, why did you want her to disappear yesterday afternoon?" In my mind, I interrogate myself ruthlessly with these questions.

Infertile parents need to somehow come to terms with ambivalence if they are to truly be freed as parents. Drawing analogies with other parts of your life can be helpful. Like, "I love my husband and we have a good marriage. Yet, last week when he came home two hours late for a special supper, I was so angry I wanted to shoot him. Does this mean I don't love him? Does this mean we shouldn't be married?" Or . . . "My mother came to visit yesterday. I love her to death, but she also drives me crazy. She implies that my house would be cleaner if I really made it a priority. Part of me wanted to never see her again because I was so upset. Does this mean we have a horrible relationship and that I don't really love her?"

I deal with these feelings toward my child on a daily basis. I love her to death, and she also drives me nuts. When she drives me nuts, I feel guilty. But in a very slow, painstaking way, I'm working away at that guilt. I've paid my dues. I waited forever to have this child. I refuse to let this legacy from infertility rob me of the full experience of parenting. I made a mistake when I vowed I would be a better than normal parent, because what my child and I both deserve is the freedom for me to be just a normal mother. Being a superparent is an expectation nobody can or should ever live up to. Instead of giving to the child and augmenting the parent, it takes away from both.

Infertility robbed me of much of the last five years of my life. I'm not going to let it have the next twenty. They belong to my daughter and me.

Suggested Reading

Glazer, Ellen Sarasohn. *The Long-Awaited Stork: A Guide to Parenting after Infertility.* New York, N.Y.: Lexington Books, 1993. Interesting guide to parenting with many anecdotes from former patients.

Simons, Harriet Fishman. *Wanting Another Child: Coping with Secondary Infertility.* New York, N.Y.: Lexington Books, 1995.

For Couples' Discussion

1. If you have no children, do you empathize with patients who have secondary infertility?

2. Are you convinced that "once we have a child, all our problems will be over"?

3. If you do conceive or adopt, will you give yourselves "permission" to be normal parents?

The noblest works and foundations
have proceeded from childless men,
which have sought to express the images of their minds
where those of their bodies have failed.

—*Francis Bacon (1561—1626)*

Chapter 16

When Resolution
Doesn't Mean Conception

Adoption

Join me [Sandi] in the first chapter of Exodus. The story begins with Pharaoh giving a command. He felt threatened by the fact that the Hebrew slaves had the Egyptians beat in both number and strength. So he gave some instructions: "Every son who is born you are to cast into the Nile, and every daughter you are to keep alive."

In the meantime, a couple from the house of Levi were married and had a daughter. Then they added a son to their family, and Pharaoh's command came as terrible news. When the baby's mother looked at her tiny child, her heart melted. She managed to hide him for three months; but when she could hide him no longer, she took a wicker basket and covered it with tar and pitch. Then she put him into it and floated it among the reeds by the bank of the Nile. His sister stood at a distance to see what would happen next.

The daughter of Pharaoh, coming to bathe in the river, brought her maidens with her. She saw the basket among the reeds and sent her maid over to fetch it. When Pharaoh's daughter opened the little bundle, she saw the child, heard him crying, and had pity on him. It didn't take long for her to figure out what had happened: "This must be one of the Hebrews' children."

The baby's sister approached her and asked, "Shall I go call a nurse for you from the Hebrew women? She could nurse the child for you."

"Yes."

So the girl went and got her mother. Then Pharaoh's daughter said to the mother, "Take this child away and nurse him for me, and I shall give you wages." So the mother took her child and cared for him.

Years passed, and after he had grown, she brought him to Pharaoh's daughter. Pharoah's daughter took him, and "he became her son" (Exod. 2:10).

I find it interesting that Scripture includes a story about a great woman who loved her child Moses, enough to make an "adoption plan" for him. This is especially relevant because we have, in our numerous contacts with potential birth mothers, encountered several pastors who have told birth mothers that "giving up your baby is wrong." Their counsel has been that "if God gifts you with a child, you are abdicating your responsibility by letting someone else raise him or her. Trust Him to provide for you." But, as Moses' mother demonstrated, sometimes you have to love someone enough to "let him or her go." In that case, she even risked sending her child to a "pagan" home to save his life.

Moses stands as an important person in the Bible who was part of an adoption arrangement. Hadassah is another: "[Mordecai] was bringing up Hadassah, that is Esther, his uncle's daughter, for she had neither father nor mother. Now the young lady was beautiful of form and face, and when her father and her mother died, Mordecai took her as his own daughter" (Esther 2:7).

In the Book of Romans we see another adoption—our own. Those who have believed in Christ are said to have received a spirit of adoption; we are also described as "waiting eagerly for our adoption as sons, the redemption of our body" (Rom. 8:15, 23). God has adopted us as His children.

My niece Devin joined our family through adoption. Her mother, my sister Mary, helped me over some of the adoption hurdles by blazing the way ahead of me. One of my great fears, which I know now to be a common one, was that I might not love an adopted child as much as I would love a biological child. Mary has experienced both adoption and birth, and she assures me that there's no difference to a mother.

"Do you love your husband?" she asks.

"Yes. He's the most important person in my life. I love him more than anybody in the whole world."

"Is he a blood relative?"

"No."

"I rest my case."

Adoption brings with it a whole new set of issues and choices, and a new cycle of hope and despair. Despair often comes and couples wonder when they'll ever have hope again. Because of the added stress, many therapists strongly recommend that couples refrain from pursuing adoption until they have completed medical treatment. There are also some important decisions to make that no one can make for you (though they may try).

During one of the first calls we received from a birth mother, the young woman told us she had some questions. We were one of five couples she wanted to meet, but she needed a decision from us first. "I want your assurance that you will take this baby—no matter what," she told us. "Before I meet you, I need that commitment from you. If the baby has genetic problems or is biracial, promise you won't back out." She already had one mentally retarded child, and because she hadn't seen the father of this child (she said she had been raped in a dark alley), she wasn't sure about race.

Much as we wanted a child, we told her no. She was asking us to immediately make a lifetime commitment to a child about whom we had only sketchy information, and the information she gave us had serious ramifications.

Later, when I talked with an adoption attorney about some of these issues, he said, "I don't understand how someone who really wants a child could say no. It makes me wonder if you're serious about adopting." Yet it was precisely because we take adoption so seriously that we had so many reservations.

Many people had said to us, "There are so many needy children out there. You'd be doing them a favor to adopt them." But the more we researched, the more we learned that perceiving ourselves as "rescuers" was one of the worst possible attitudes we could have. Adopting a child is a blessing. Those who perceive themselves as "doing someone a favor" are not ready to adopt. Pity is such an insult. When making a lifetime commitment to someone, it's no time to let guilt or excessive altruism take over.

We had given racial issues a lot of thought. In fact, in a later adoption possibility we said yes to a biracial situation. We do believe all children are special and created in God's image, regardless of race, age, nationality, or limitation. We also believe there is no room for racial discrimination in the lives of God's people.

If God is nudging you to welcome an older child, a child from another nation, a child with special needs, and/or a child of another race into your family, no doubt He has great blessings in store for you. But make that choice because you want to, not because you "have" to. Couples who have endured infertility's losses must recognize the additional challenges involved in these choices and embrace them willingly.

In her book *Adopting after Infertility,* author Pat Johnston identifies infertility's six losses: (1) loss of control, (2) loss of individual genetic continuity, (3) loss of a jointly conceived child, (4) loss of the pregnancy and birth experiences, (5) loss of emotional expectations surrounding pregnancy and birth, and (6) loss of an opportunity to nurture and parent a new generation. Of these six, adoption is the "cure" for only the last one—the opportunity to nurture and parent a new generation.

With some choices, adoption actually adds to this list: (1) loss of privacy about your infertility for the rest of your life, as is the case when you adopt a child whose race or nationality prompts people to ask, (2) loss of a child who "looks like you," as is the case in transracial and some international adoptions, (3) loss of a lifestyle in which all family members are healthy, and/or (4) loss of the experience of parenting a newborn, as is the case with adopting an older child. Only you and your spouse can decide how important these are for you.

However, the adoption route may not be for you. It's not for everyone, or maybe you've been riding that bumpy road long enough to decide you want to look at another option. Whatever your circumstances, choosing to live childfree may be a better option for you.

Choosing Childfree

The Texas life insurance company where I worked for nine years was bought by a company in Atlanta, and five hundred of us were slated for layoff. I felt really upset until I was offered a job with the new company in Atlanta. Once I chose not to take it, I felt differently about losing my job. The outcome was the same—unemployment—but the fact that I had been allowed to make the choice changed my outlook.

Having the freedom to make a choice affects our viewpoint. That's why it's important, at some point, to make a conscious decision to live without children rather than to passively feel victimized for the rest of your life. If you want a child, there are usually ways around the obstacles. If you don't plan to adopt after ending medical treatment, consider making an active point-in-time choice rather than coasting along in indecision and uncertainty forever.

Most couples who have actively chosen this option prefer to call themselves "childfree" rather than "childless." "Childfree" emphasizes wholeness, fulfillment, and completeness rather than the absence of something. Viewing one's self as having moved from the first label to the latter is actually a moment of resolution.

That's not to say we ever reach a moment in time after which we never look back. "As complex as human beings are, this kind of resolution is certainly an unrealistic expectation," say obstetrician Jean Carter and her professor husband Michael. They believe that making the decision to become childfree is a process of reaching relative peace about the decision.

Jean and Michael became my friends through a national support group. They describe the decision-making process they went through in deciding to live childfree in their excellent book, *Sweet Grapes: How to Stop Being Infertile and Start Living Again*. Now, years after writing their book, they verify that their decision has become even more "durable" with passing time.

For some, the idea that a couple who has felt desperate to have a child would somehow find themselves actually embracing such a choice may seem incomprehensible, but the decision comes slowly. It usually comes near the end of the grief cycle, and it comes at a time when it has been made clear that children will not come biologically. Other alternatives begin to look more interesting, even appealing. The advantages in the tragedy begin to emerge. One of the benefits of being unable to fulfill the commandment, "Be fruitful and multiply," is more freedom to concentrate instead on another commandment, "make disciples."

Christian writer and speaker Jeanne Hendricks has said a common thread that runs through every woman is the need to nurture, but that doesn't necessarily mean she needs to be a biological mother: "Get it out of your head that being a mother is having a baby," she says. "Being a mother in the Christian sense of the word is passing along a message. It's much more than physical. It's a spiritual, emotional, and total impact process. It's my giving of everything that I've got to the next generation because that's the way God intended it."

In her book, *Childless Is Not Less,* Vicky Love points to Priscilla and Aquila, a New Testament couple, as models. Because of the freedom they enjoyed in having few family responsibilities, Priscilla and Aquila had the opportunity to play key roles in the lives of the apostle Paul and Apollos, strong leaders in the emerging church.

Love, who has served for years with her husband as a missionary in Mexico City, writes, "What a glad relief came to my own heart to realize that I had been patterning my longing for life after the wrong model. For years everyone tried to encourage us in the same unreproductive direction, commenting: 'You would be such great parents.' 'Remember Sarah. Don't ever give up hope' 'Why don't you adopt?' There never were any adequate answers. I now realize that those of us who are childfree do not have to become Abrahams and Sarahs. There are Pauls, Johns, and Annas; Mary-Martha-and-Lazaruses; and there are Priscillas and Aquilas in God's ample and varied pattern book."[1]

One question couples without children wrestle with is, "Who will take care of me in my old age? What if I end up alone?" An obituary in a missions newsletter answered that question for me.

I never knew Grace Anderson, but she had lived to be ninety-two years old, it said. She and her sister had gone to Guatemala to work as missionaries, and there Grace had married a widower with two daughters. They went on to have two more daughters together.

Grace served the Lord for another thirty-five years after her husband's death. The write-up said she enjoyed retirement among family and friends in California. Then, ten years before her death, she moved to a Christian retirement village in Oklahoma, far from her family.

It was the final line that grabbed me: "A number of missions retirees and other friends ministered to her until she slipped into the Lord's presence."

Grace had raised four children. Had they been her primary caretakers in the last ten years? No. But God's family had been there to minister to her.

That obituary answers the question in two ways. First, it serves as a reminder that having biological children is no guarantee that they'll be either willing or able to be caretakers. Second, it reminds us that like the birds of the air, we are known to the Lord, and He Himself will care for us if we "seek first the kingdom of God." He may use our biological or our spiritual family to do so, or maybe both.

Some who choose to live childfree find themselves constantly explaining that their choice is not a rejection of adoption. When most members of the infertility support network have chosen adoption, it can feel like a choice to set themselves apart from friends. Others often fail to understand such a decision because it differs from how they feel or see things. Childfree is not a rejection of adoption; it's just a different way of resolving infertility. Others believe a decision not to adopt means you're "stuck on genetics" but love has little to do with genetics. As one childfree woman explains, "Adopting a child requires and brings with it a completely different attitude than conceiving one." We must have the grace to allow for differing viewpoints.

Does childfree mean you have to have a glamorous career? No. Several women I know who have chosen this option spend their days at home. Their time is devoted to people and interesting pursuits.

Can a couple really be happy without children? Only the two of you can answer this question for yourselves, but studies on marriage indicate that the happiest couples do not necessarily raise children together. The important factor is not whether a couple has children, but whether they agree children should or should not be part of their lives together.

Is a childfree choice a selfish one? Some would say so, and the answer here is that it can be. So can a life of parenting. Selfishness is revealed not in the number or lack of children but in the lifestyle. Lauren, who is trying to decide whether to remain childfree writes, "If I had children, I'd probably quit my job—a job that lets me nurture and assist dozens of college students through their academic careers. At graduation I had three different students tell me they couldn't have made it without me. Is it selfish not to want to give this up? Lately, we've been talking about doing missionary work in Eastern Europe, an option we wouldn't have even considered if we had kids."

Last fall, as Gary and I stood in a chapel in Northleach, England, a memorial engraved in stone on one of the walls caught my eye. It said, "In memory of Mary Glover, died 1782. Age sixty-eight, who having no children or next of kin, adopted the people of this parish and left a handsome endowment for an alms house for aged men having no pension. This with her charity renders her the greatest benefactress to this town. Hereto recorded in her memory to encourage others do likewise."

Can people with no children leave a lasting legacy? Yes.

Is childfree a valid option? Of course.

Is it biblical? Certainly. The Bible is filled with characters who lived full lives without children—the Son of God being one of them. Is it popular? Well, no. But in the words of Robert Frost:

I shall be telling this with a sigh
Somewhere ages and ages hence;
Two roads diverged in a wood and I,
I took the one less traveled by,
And that has made the difference.[2]

Adoption Resources

Adoptive Families of America
800/372-3300
> National organization that provides information and support groups.

American Academy of Adoption Attorneys
P.O. Box 33053
Washington, DC 20033

National association of adoption lawyers; provides directory of attorneys by state.

Families for Private Adoption
202/722-0338
Provides support, education, and publications for those interested in private adoption.

International Concerns Committee for Children
303/494-8333
Provides information on international adoption.

National Adoption Foundation
203/791-3811
Provides needs-based grants to prospective adoptive parents.

National Adoption Information Clearinghouse
301/231-6512
Specializes in information and advocacy for placement of older and special needs children; provides newsletter.

National Council for Adoption
202/328-1200
Organization of nonprofit adoption agencies. Promotes sound adoption practices. Serves as clearinghouse for adoption information.

North American Council on Adoptable Children
612/644-3036
Specializes in information and advocacy for placement of older and special needs children.

Over-40 Adoption Directory
813/983-8360
Directory for prospective adoptive parents over age forty.

Perspectives Press
P.O. Box 90318
Indianapolis, IN 46290-0318
317/872-3055
Publishes books on infertility and adoption only.

The National Adoption Assistance Training, Resource and Information Network (NAA-TRIN) is a network that can provide state-specific fact sheets on subsidized adoption topics, including special needs definitions, notification practices, benefit offerings, and fair hearing procedures. The hotline number is 800/470-6665.

Tapestry Books
http://www.webcom.com/~tapestry/
This site on the World Wide Web has a huge selection of books on adoption and infertility.

Suggested Reading on Childfree Living

Love, Vicky. *Childless Is Not Less.* Minneapolis, Minn.: Bethany House Publishers, 1984.

Carter, Jean, M.D., and Michael Carter, Ph.D., *Sweet Grapes: How to Stop Being Infertile and Start Living Again.* (Indianapolis, Ind.: Perspectives Press, 1989). An excellent guide to thinking through the decision to live childfree.

Organization for Couples Choosing to Live Childfree
Childfree Network
7777 Sunrise Boulevard Suite 1800
Citrus Heights, CA 95610
916/773-7178

Questions for Couples' Discussion

The options of adoption and childfree living require much thought and communication. Entire books have been written on both subjects and the decision-making processes involved. The questions here serve as a starting point, but we urge you to investigate further, starting with the resources listed.

1. Which of the losses related to fertility are the most difficult for you to accept? Is the same true for your spouse?

2. Of the two options, adoption and childfree living, which appeals more to you and why?

3. Why do you want to have children?

4. Are you willing to end treatment if and when the time comes to pursue adoption?

5. Is the adoption of a child with special needs an option for you? Why or why not? Are you both in agreement here? Do others pressure you to consider adoption scenarios with which you are uncomfortable?

6. What are the advantages and disadvantages of choosing a childfree lifestyle?

Epilogue

*I*f Mother's Day in America is a big deal, Mother's Day in Culiacan, Sinaloa, Mexico, is *huge*. I know because I experienced it firsthand.

Dr. Bill had asked us months ago to accompany him on another mission trip. He wanted to take a team to help a church in Mexico.

The physical needs of the people in the colony of Felipe Angeles—especially hunger—overwhelmed me, but I was even more amazed at the spiritual hunger. We spent our mornings walking door-to-door, sharing with those who wanted to hear. Every home I visited saw at least one profession of faith. The people responded enthusiastically to the message of God's love and grace, opening their hearts and homes to the Lord and to us.

In a little shack, I found a woman at home who told me Mother's Day was Wednesday (a surprise to me) and asked if I had children. When I told her that they were all with Jesus, tears rolled down her cheeks. This woman had almost nothing, and I had so much, but she was still filled with compassion for me.

I awoke Wednesday morning: Mother's Day in Mexico. A national holiday. Mothers had been serenaded at midnight. Tonight there would be a special church celebration. School would be canceled for the day. Offices would be closed.

I looked at the clock: 5:00 A.M. My stomach ached. "Oh, God, don't let me be sick. I've come all this way to do a work. Please let me go out today!" I begged. Several hours later, Dr. Bill gave me some medication. Probably because my helper didn't show combined with the fact that I still looked a little under the weather, Dr. Bill had me spend the morning with him. I felt weak but I was well enough to go. As we walked along the dirt road, we came upon two men sitting in the shade. They were in their mid-forties. One told us he was a secondary school teacher enjoying his Mother's Day holiday off from work. So there I stood, a woman who generally hates Mother's Day. Later, I had to acknowledge that this man, who was moved to tears by our message, would not have been there had it not been for all the hoopla about Mother's Day. When we finished, the two men expressed their desire to begin a personal relationship with Christ. Then the teacher said, "This is a very important message for my family." The other agreed.

That night, Dr. Bill preached the Mother's Day sermon. He pointed out that Mother's Day is hard for a lot of people—for those who have lost mothers, for those who have lost children, for those who cannot be mothers for whatever reason, and for those who are estranged from their mothers or children. I looked down my row, and every person was crying. There was the man whose mother died twenty years ago. Next, there was a woman whose mother rejected her when she married a Christian. Then there was me. On my other side sat a young woman, recently married, who wanted children yesterday, but she has agreed with her husband to wait until he finishes school. In front of me sat a single woman who wants to marry, but her previous boyfriend had told her when he proposed that he didn't want children, and that price had been too high for her to pay.

I wept. I wept for our empty cradle. But even more, I felt the pain of those around me, and I hurt for the mothers I had seen all day who were struggling so hard to feed their children.

Dr. Bill continued, exhorting the women to serve the Lord as unique creations of God in their homes, but also to reproduce in another dimension. I thought of Lucy and my first trip to the former USSR, when I saw the reality of spiritual reproduction in such a powerful way.

One of the Mexican church's female leaders reached out to touch me. Later she told me kindly but earnestly through a translator, "Don't weep for your children; weep for our people." At one time her words would have hurt. But not now. I knew it was OK to weep for both.

At the end of the service, the men presented each woman with a carnation—just one. But Mike, one of the guys on my team who knew the pain of pregnancy loss, walked over to me, burst into tears, and shoved four carnations into my open palm.

I have a lot of joy in my life. I would describe my life now as abundant, but we have no neat package tied up with a pretty bow to show off as the "grand finale" to our infertility. At this point, we still don't know how or when it will all end; but after going through the grief process for ten years, we are seeing that even without a happy conclusion, we can reach the "resolution" stage. As we try to make plans for the future, we are finding ways to live "today" to the fullest, taking one day at a time.

I heard of a missionary who was moved to a new post. A native with whom he had worked wanted to make him a gift. He carved an intricate wooden cross, but he was unable to complete it before the missionary moved up the mountain. So the native made the several-day walk to present it to him. Upon receiving the gift, the missionary felt overwhelmed. He exclaimed, "I feel so unworthy to accept this; it's so beautiful, and you've come so far to get here." The friend replied, "But you must accept it! The journey was part of the gift."

And so it is with infertility. When we stand before the throne of the One we love but have not seen—the One who first loved us—we will receive crowns of reward; but rather than wearing them on our heads, we will spontaneously cast them at His feet in worship. And our treacherous journey, if we have traveled it well, will greatly add to the preciousness of our gift.

Bill's Finale: The Laughter and Tears

Another day at the office. But now, after these months of writing, the office door says "Pastor's Study" instead of "Doctor's Office." Now the appointment schedule is full of spiritual needs and counseling opportunities. My study time is in God's Word instead of journals of advancing medical technology. What an incredible journey these months have been as this life change unfolded.

I experienced so many changes. My life work has moved from concentration on the "natural" birth to spiritual birth. What a privilege to have both experiences in one lifetime. I see so many similarities between pastoral ministry and being an Ob/Gyn physician. (I am still a licensed medical doctor; I just don't practice medicine as an occupation any longer.)

Looking back, I can see the hand of the Lord in all of it. When I first came to know Jesus Christ, I was a freshman in college. I felt a strong calling into pastoral ministry at that time but didn't know where to turn. None of my friends and few in my family could envision me as anything other than a physician, since that is all I had ever wanted to be.

I returned to my premed education, went to medical school, and became a doctor. I loved the work and the people. I pursued my specialty training in Ob/Gyn, completed my training, and began private practice. The Lord provided a place to work, and my practice grew.

During that time and due to the proximity of Dallas Theological Seminary to my office, I had the privilege of caring for many patients from the seminary student body and faculty staff wives. Many great theological discussions during labor and delivery reminded me of my commitment to God and His calling on my life. I enrolled in seminary, planning to take night courses to improve my skills as a Sunday school teacher and, perhaps, open some doors for mission-ary involvement. I never imagined God would consider "reclaiming" me at this stage of my life for full-time service.

I loved medicine, and, moreover, I loved the patient and family contact. I could see no way of ever leaving obstetrics. I knew in the privacy of my prayer closet that God had spe-cial plans, as I believe He does for everyone. Yet I was reluc-tant. Then, after I had enjoyed forty years of excellent health, including running many marathons, my wife detected a new heart murmur which would prove to be a crucial turning point. Almost immediately I was forced to give up the practice of obstetrics and have my heart valve surgically repaired. Interestingly, from the standpoint of God's sovereignty, I was nearing the completion of my sem-inary degree.

My heart surgery went great. My patients showed their support with calls, cards, and letters. I was and remain deeply grateful. I wanted to return to full-time practice as soon as possible. It didn't work out quite that way, however. Irregular heart rhythms postoperatively required rest and medications that made all-night obstetric and emergency room shifts impossible.

I had been active on cross-cultural mission trips prior to surgery and had been helping out as pulpit-supply thor-oughly expecting to carry on some bivocational type of min-istry. Then I came to Wildwood Baptist Church in Mesquite, Texas. This church had as its interim pastor a friend of mine whose full-time job often required him to be out of town. He asked if I could fill in for him occasionally and I gladly accepted. Over the course of several months, I fell in love with Wildwood and God confirmed in my heart, as well as through others, that this was the place for me. This church needed a full-time pastor, not a bivocational one, and they asked if I would be willing to leave medicine to serve here. I knew, perhaps before they did, that this was what God had been preparing me for. So with a mixture of joy and sadness, I closed the doors of my medical office and began a new ministry.

In these pages, you have seen selected experiences from over fifteen years in medicine recalled, reviewed, and recorded to illustrate the depth of my patients' burdens. I am especially grateful to those many patients who allowed us to share their personal struggles. I was touched by their willingness and candor expressed in the hopes that others might benefit from their experiences. My life is so much the richer for having known each of these families; and during the process of writing, it was a joy to recall so many fine memories.

As I move on from medicine, I must applaud the diligent and often heroic efforts on the part of the infertility patients and the medical personnel that render their care. Indeed, most of my friends and colleagues who have devoted their lives to infertility care are men and women of great integrity and compassion. I will miss the camaraderie we shared as we worked together for a common cause. Most of all, I dearly miss the patients, the lives and trials we shared, the laughter and the tears.

Sandi and I have been riders together on the infertility roller coaster. We have also walked the streets of Belarus, Ukraine, and Mexico, sharing the gospel together, watching the Lord draw souls to Himself; on this project we have agonized over each section, praying that it would honor God and encourage the readers. Our desire is that those who read this, whether they be patients, health-care people, or pastoral folks, will be challenged to a deeper sensitivity and understanding of the many complex issues involved.

I have learned so much about the emotional battles and deep personal needs behind the medical maze. I trust that this book, while not providing all the answers, will at least give voice and comfort to the many silent sufferers as well as helpful direction to the caregivers. My prayer is that God, who is sufficient for all our needs, will meet people in their hearts and minister His grace to each spirit.

Appendix

RESOLVE
National Office
1310 Broadway, Somerville, MA 02144-1731
Business Office 617/623-1156   *Fax* 617/623-0252

Local Chapter Contact List

RESOLVE's volunteer-run chapters offer many services to members. Please call the chapter or site nearest you.

Resolve of Alaska*
P.O. Box 243234
Anchorage, AK 99524
907-566-0022

Resolve of Northwest Arkansas*
P.O. Box 4492
Fayetteville, AR 72702
501-444-2186; 800-568-0814

Resolve of Tucson, Arizona*
11909 Copper Butte Dr.
Tucson, AZ 85737
602-742-0863

Resolve of Valley of the Sun, Arizona*
P.O. Box 54214
Phoenix, AZ 85078
602-995-3933

Resolve of Greater San Diego, California*
P.O. Box 15982
San Diego, CA 92175-0785
619-595-3988

Resolve of Greater Los Angeles, California*
P.O. Box 15344
Los Angeles, CA 90015
310-326-2630

Resolve of Northern California*
312 Sutter St., 6th Floor
San Francisco, CA 94108
415-459-2995, 788-6772, Fax 788-6774

Resolve of Orange County, California
P.O. Box 50693
Irvine, CA 92619-0693
714-859-0580

Resolve of Colorado*
P.O. Box 61096
Denver, CO 80206
303-469-5261

Resolve of Fairfield County, Connecticut
P.O. Box 16763
Stamford, CT 06905-6763
203-329-1147

Resolve of Greater Hartford, Connecticut
P.O. Box 370083
West Hartford, CT 06137-0083
203-523-8337

Resolve of Washington DC Metro Area
P.O. Box 2038
Washington, DC 20013-2038
202-362-5555

Resolve of Ft. Lauderdale, Florida*
1401 NE 9th St. #9
Fort Lauderdale, FL 33304-4410
305-749-9500

Resolve of the Palm Beaches, Florida*
20423 State Rd. 7, Suite 247
Boca Raton, FL 33498
407-731-5930

Resolve of Georgia
Box 343, 2480-4 Briarcliff Rd.
Atlanta, GA 30329
404-233-8443

Resolve of Hawaii*
P.O. Box 29193
Honolulu, HI 96820
808-528-8559

Resolve of Idaho
c/o Women's Life
103 W. State
Boise, ID 83702
208-386-3033

Resolve of Illinois*
318 Half Day Road #300
Buffalo Grove, IL 60089-6547
312-743-1623; 1-800-395-5522

Resolve of Indiana*
6103 Ashway Court
Indianapolis, IN 46224
317-767-5999

Resolve of Kansas City, Missouri*
P.O. Box 414603
Kansas City, MO 64141
913-791-2432; 913-648-2892

Resolve of Kentucky*
P.O. Box 22825
Lexington, KY 40522-2825
502-589-4313; 606-281-4603

Resolve of Louisiana
4610 Anson St.
New Orleans, LA 70131
504-454-6987

Resolve of the Bay State, Massachusetts*
P.O. Box 1553
Waltham, MA 02254-1553
617-647-1614, Fax 617-899-7207

Resolve of Maryland
P.O. Box 5664
Baltimore, MD 21210
410-243-0235

Resolve of Maine*
P.O. Box 10691
Portland, ME 04104
207-774-4357; 207-945-7598

Resolve of Michigan*
P.O. Box 2185
Southfield, MI 48037
810-680-0093

Resolve of Twin Cities, Minnesota*
1313 Fifth St., SE, Ste. 120A
Minneapolis, MN 55414
612-379-3882

Resolve of St. Louis, Missouri
P.O. Box 131
Hazelwood, MO 63042
314-968-6504

Resolve of Triangle, North Carolina
P.O. Box 5564
Cary, NC 27511
919-477-2360

Resolve of Nebraska*
P.O. Box 24527
Omaha, NE 68124-0527
402-449-6875

Resolve of New Hampshire*
12 Bayshore Drive
Greenland, NH 03840-2204
603-427-0410

Resolve of New Jersey*
P.O. Box 4335
Warren, NJ 07059-0335
908-679-7171

Resolve of New Mexico*
8100 Mountain Rd., NE, Suite 204B
Albuquerque, NM 87108
505-266-1170; 524-1489

Resolve of Northern Nevada
P.O. Box 9749
Reno, NV 89507-9749
702-852-3205

Resolve of Capital District, New York
P.O. Box 12901
Albany, NY 12212
518-464-3848

Resolve of Long Island, New York*
P.O. Box 516
Plainview, NY 11803
516-649-7034

Resolve of New York City, Staten Island
718-983-8202

Resolve of New York City*
P.O. Box 185
Gracie Station, NY 10028
212-764-0802

Resolve of New York City, Westchester
914-664-3009

Resolve of Ohio*
P.O. Box 141277
Columbus, OH 43214-6277
1-800-414-Ohio

Resolve of Oklahoma
P.O. Box 549
Okarche, OK 73762-0549
918-621-5250; 405-949-8857

Resolve of Oregon*
P.O. Box 40717
Portland, OR 97240
503-762-0449

Resolve of Pittsburgh, Pennsylvania
P.O. Box 11203
Pittsburgh, PA 15238
412-921-3501

Resolve of Southcentral Pennsylvania Area
P.O. Box 402
Camp Hill, PA 17011
717-234-8583

Resolve of Philadelphia, Pennsylvania,
P.O. Box 0215
Merion Station, PA 19066-0215
215-849-3920

Resolve of the Ocean State, Rhode Island
P.O. Box 28201
Providence, RI 02908
401-421-4695

Resolve of Upstate South Carolina
204 Fernbrook Circle
Spartanburg, SC 29307-2966
803-542-9092

Resolve of Tennessee
4770 Germantown Road, Ext., Ste. 327
Memphis, TN 38141
901-541-5360

Resolve of Central Texas
P.O. Box 49783
Austin, TX 78765
512-453-2171

Resolve of Dallas/Ft. Worth, Texas
3100 Creek Crossing
Mesquite, TX 75181-1526
214-621-7560

Resolve of Houston, Texas
P.O. Box 441212
Houston, TX 77244-1212
713-975-5324

Resolve of South Texas*
P.O. Box 380223
San Antonio, TX 78280
210-492-5142

Resolve of Utah
P.O. Box 57531
Salt Lake City, UT 84157-0531
801-483-4024

Resolve of Virginia*
P.O. Box 70372
Richmond, VA 23255-0372
804-751-5761; 804-459-5856

Resolve of Vermont*
P.O. Box 4431
Burlington, VT 05406
802-657-2542

Resolve of Washington State*
P.O. Box 31231
Seattle, WA 98103-1231
206-524-7257; 509-535-9361

Resolve of Wisconsin*
P.O. Box 23406
Milwaukee, WI 53223
414-521-4590; 608-231-9955

[*] Chapter with more than one meeting site.

If there is not a chapter in your region, you may wish to contact the national office about the informal member-to-member medical contact system.

Notes

Chapter 1

1. John and Sylvia Van Regenmorter and Joe McIlhaney, M.D., *Dear God, Why Can't We Have a Baby?* (Grand Rapids, Mich.: Baker Book House, 1986), 69.

2. Joe McIlhaney, M.D., *1,250 Healthcare Questions Women Ask.* (Grand Rapids, Mich.: Baker Book House, 1988), 503.

3. Larry Greil, "Infertility: His and Hers," RESOLVE of Kansas City, (September 1991)., 3.

4. Richard Krusen, Ph.D., "Infertility and Men," RESOLVE of Dallas/Fort Worth (April/May 1992), 8.

5. Linda Smith Hellmann, LCSW-C, "Infertility and My Spouse!" RESOLVE of Maryland (Spring/Summer 1995).

6. Jan Short, "Infertility Tales," *Self* magazine (April 1990).

7. Griel, "Infertility: His and Hers."

8. Willard F. Harley, Jr. *His Needs, Her Needs* (Grand Rapids, Mich.: Fleming Revell, 1986), 10.

9. Delores Steinhauser, "A Message for Husbands," RESOLVE of Orange County (June 1994), 3.

10. As reported by Carol A. McDonald, in her seminar titled, "Women and Men Working Together in Management," delivered at Christian Management Institute, Dallas, Texas.

11. Robert Kohn, "Patterns of Hemispheric Specialization in Pre-Schoolers," *Neuropsychologia*, vol. 12:505–12. As reported in *The Language of Love* by Gary Smalley and John Trent, Ph.D., chapter 4.

12. J. Levy, "The Adaptive Advantages of Cerebral Asymmetry and Communication," *Annals of the New York Academy of Sciences*, vol. 229:264–72. As reported in *The Language of Love* by Gary Smalley and John Trent, Ph.D., chapter 4.

13. As reported by Carol A. McDonald, in her seminar titled, "Women and Men Working Together in Management," delivered at Christian Management Institute, Dallas, Texas.

14. Merle Bombardieri, "The Twenty Minute Rule: First Aid for Couples in Distress," National RESOLVE Newsletter (December 1983), 5.

15. Tami Steele. From RESOLVE of Dallas/Fort Worth (January-February 1990), 8.

Chapter 2

1. R. M. Sabatellil, R. L. Meth, and S. M. Gavazzi, "Factors mediating the adjustment to involuntary childlessness," *Family Relations*, (1988), 37, 338-43. The men in this study were, in general, responding to their spouse's infertile condition (only 7 of the 29 males had been treated for infertility problems).

2. Vicky Love, *Childless Is Not Less* (Minneapolis, Minn.: Bethany House Publishers, 1984), 80.

3. W. Andrew Hoffecker, "Prenatal Techniques," *Tabletalk* (September 1994), 8.

4. Beth Spring, *The Infertile Couple* (Elgin, Ill.: David C. Cook Publishing Co., 1987), 51.

5. Sabatellil, Meth, and Gavazzi, *op. cit.*

6. Sally Squires, "Sex Therapy—Helping Couples Achieve Intimacy," *Washington Post* (30 July 1986), 13.

7. Ellen Sarasohn Glazer and Susan Lewis Cooper, *Without Child* (Lexington, Mass.: Lexington Press, 1988), 3.

8. Arthur Ralston, "She's Not Having a Baby," *GQ* (September 1989), 281.

9. Susan Morley, "A Qualitative Study of Infertility Resolution," RESOLVE of the Bay State (May 1994), 7.

10. Linda Hellmann, LCSW, "Sex and Romance in the Land of Infertility: How to Have Two Sex Lives without Having an Affair," RESOLVE of Dallas/Fort Worth (Feb./March 92).

11. Elisa Morgan, *I'm Tired of Waiting* (Wheaton, Ill.: Victor Books, 1989), 69.

Chapter 3

1. R. M. Sabatelli, R. L. Meth, and S. M. Gavazzi, "Factors mediating the adjustment to involuntary childlessness," *Family Relations* (1988), 37, 338-343.

2. Colleen Botsios, "Julia Child . . . less," RESOLVE of Dallas/Fort Worth (January-February, 1990).

Chapter 4

1. Aline Zoldbrod, Ph.D., "Grieving and Coping: On the Need to Deal with Stress Differently During Different Stages of Fertility Treatment," RESOLVE of Dallas/Fort Worth, (February/March 1994).

2. Isabel Kuhn, *Green Leaf in Drought* (OMF Books: Singapore, 1958).

3. Mary Martin Mason, *The Miracle Seekers: An Anthology of Infertility* (Fort Wayne, Ind.: Perspectives Press, 1987), 39.

4. Elizabeth Elliot, *Let Me Be a Woman* (Wheaton, Ill.: Tyndale House Publishers, Inc., 1976), 42.

Chapter 5

1. Lisa Foster, "Don't Let the Lights Go Out," RESOLVE of Pittsburgh (Holiday 1992), 4.

Chapter 6

1. Jody Earle, "Choosing a Doctor and a Coat," RESOLVE of Central New York (Fall 1988).

2. As reported in *USA Today* (25, January 1995), 6D.

Chapter 7

1. Kim Yankee, RESOLVE of the Washington Metropolitan Area Newsletter (January 1987).

2. Dr. Dan Allender and Dr. Tremper Longman, *Cry of the Soul: How our Emotions Reveal our Deepest Questions about God* (Colorado Springs, Colo.: NavPress, 1994), 36–37.

3. Richard J. Foster, *Prayer: Finding the Heart's True Home* (San Francisco: HarperCollins, 1992), 23.

4. Neil Clark Warren, Ph.D., *Make Anger Your Ally* (Focus on the Family: Colorado Springs, Colo.: 1990), n.p.

5. Eugene Peterson, *Under the Unpredictable Plant: An Exploration in Vocational Holiness* (Grand Rapids, Mich.: William B. Eerdmans Publishing Company, 1992), 101.

Chapter 8

1. Michael Gold, *Without Child* (Lexington, Mass.: Lexington Books, 1988), 75.

2. For a detailed biblical explanation of the purpose of mankind, consult John Piper's book, *Desiring God.*

3. C. S. Lewis. *The Great Divorce* (New York: Macmillan Publishing Co., Inc., 1946), 126–127.

4. Rev. William Wolkovich, *Human Development,* vol. 15, no. 3 (Fall 1994), 38.

Chapter 9

1. Sue Bohlin, RESOLVE of Dallas/Fort Worth, (December 92/January 93), 4.

2. Andrea Stephens, *Focus on the Family,* "Babyless" (November 1994).

3. Betsy McClung, "A Faith Born Out of Emotional Trauma," *Pittsburgh Post-Gazette,* (3 November 1984).

4. Philip Yancey, *Disappointment with God* (Grand Rapids, Mich.: Zondervan Publishing House, 1988). Text from cover jacket.

Chapter 10

1. Barbara Eck Menning, *Infertility: A Guide for Childless Couples* (New York, N.Y.: Prentice Hall, 1988), 97.

2. Dr. John Martin, an adoptive father, has written an excellent series on 1 and 2 Samuel in the theological journal, *Bibliotheca Sacra.*

3. Roy Zuck, *Basic Bible Interpretation* (Wheaton, Ill.: Victor Books, 1991), 131–132.

4. *Basic Care Booklet 19: Questions and Answers on Infertility and Birth Control.* Medical Training Institute of America (1994), 7, 8.

5. See note on 1 Samuel 1:2 in *The Ryrie Study Bible.*

6. Michael Gold, *And Hannah Wept: Infertility, Adoption and the Jewish Couple* (New York, N.Y.: Jewish Publication Society, 1988), 69.

7. Jean Gilroy, "When Childlessness Becomes Faithlessness," RESOLVE of New York City Newsletter (March 1992), 2.

Chapter 11

1. Data from a 1995 report in *Fertility and Sterility* 64, 13–21.

2. *Op cit.*

Chapter 12

1. Brian Calhoun, M.D., *When a Husband Is Infertile* (Grand Rapids, Mich.: Baker Book House, 1994), 92–93.

2. John Van Regenmorter and Sylvia and Joe McIlhaney, M.D., *Dear God, Why Can't We Have a Baby?* (Grand Rapids, Mich.: Baker Book House), 121.

3. W. Andrew Hoffecker in "Prenatal Techniques," *Tabletalk* (September 1994), 8.

4. Kirby Anderson, brochure on "Artificial Reproduction," Probe Ministries, 1993.

5. R. Ruth Barton, *Becoming a Woman of Strength* (Wheaton: Harold Shaw Publishers), 161.

6. Debra Evans, *Without Moral Limits*, 121.

7. Phil Brewster, "Donor Kid Dad," RESOLVE of Northern California (May/June 1995), 7.

8. Susan Cooper and Ellen Sarasohn Glazer, eds., *Without Child: Experiencing and Resolving Infertility* (Lexington, Mass.: Lexington Books, D.C. Health, 1988), 121.

9. Joe McIlhaney, M.D., *Dear God, Why Can't We Have a Baby?* 121.

10. Margaret Brown, "My Turn: Whose Eyes Are These, Whose Nose?" *Newsweek* (7 March 1994), 12.

11. From RESOLVE of New York City (March 1988).

12. Mike Mason, *The Mystery of Marriage* (Sisters, Oreg.: Multnomah Books, 1985).

Chapter 15

1. Daniel Rosen, RESOLVE of Greater Los Angeles Newsletter (Spring 1994).

Chapter 16

1. Vicky Love, *Childless Is Not Less* (Minneapolis, Minn.: Bethany House Publishers, 1984), 180.

2. From Robert Frost's "The Road Not Taken."